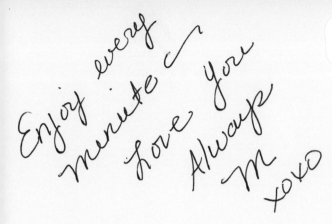

Enjoy every
minute ⌒
Love You
Always
M
xoxo

The New Rules of Pregnancy

The New Rules of Pregnancy

What to eat, do,
think about, and let
go of while your body
is making a baby

**ADRIENNE L. SIMONE, MD, JAQUELINE WORTH, MD,
AND DANIELLE CLARO**

Photographs by Winky Lewis

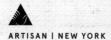

ARTISAN | NEW YORK

Library of Congress Cataloging-in-Publication Data
Names: Simone, Adrienne L., author. | Worth, Jaqueline, author. | Claro, Danielle, author.
Title: The new rules of pregnancy : Adrienne L. Simone, MD, Jaqueline Worth, MD, and Danielle Claro ; photographs by Winky Lewis.
Description: New York : Artisan, a division of Workman Publishing Co., Inc., 2019.
Identifiers: LCCN 2018039172 | ISBN 9781579658571 (hardcover : alk. paper)
Subjects: LCSH: Pregnancy—Popular works. | Pregnancy—Nutritional aspects—Popular works. | Pregnancy—Psychological aspects—Popular works.
Classification: LCC RG560 .S56 2019 | DDC 618.2/42—dc23
LC record available at https://lccn.loc.gov/2018039172

Design by Renata Di Biase

Artisan books are available at special discounts when purchased in bulk for premiums and sales promotions as well as for fund-raising or educational use. Special editions or book excerpts also can be created to specification. For details, contact the Special Sales Director at the address below, or send an e-mail to specialmarkets@workman.com.

For speaking engagements, contact speakersbureau@workman.com.

Published by Artisan
A division of Workman Publishing Co., Inc.
225 Varick Street
New York, NY 10014-4381
artisanbooks.com

Artisan is a registered trademark of Workman Publishing Co., Inc.

Published simultaneously in Canada by Thomas Allen & Son, Limited

Printed in China

First printing, February 2019

1 3 5 7 9 10 8 6 4 2

What's magical, sometimes, has
deeper roots than reason.

—*Mary Oliver*

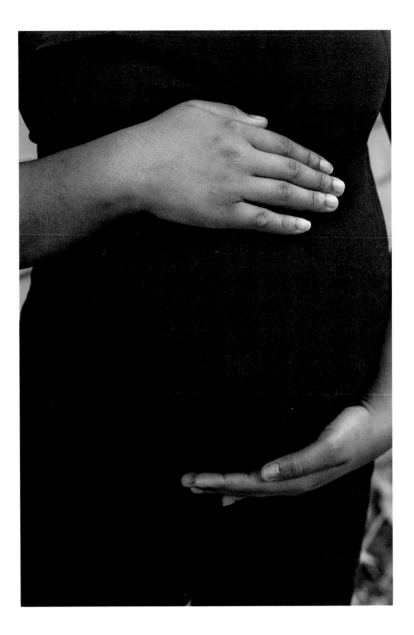

CONTENTS

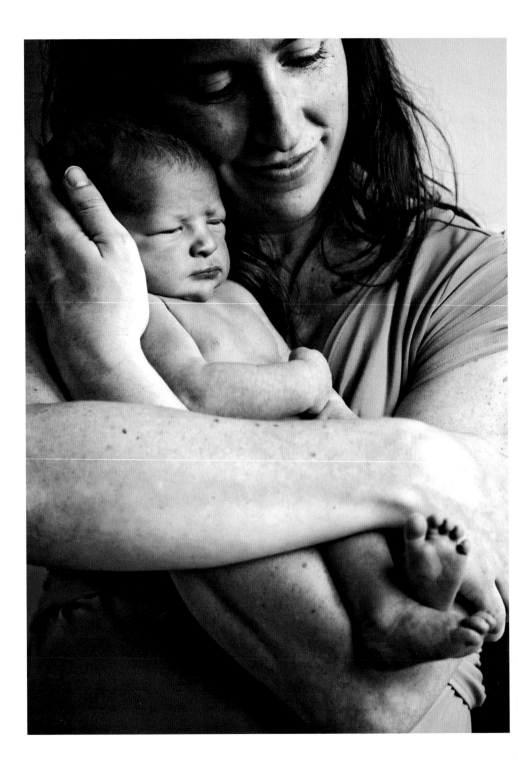

THE BIG PICTURE

Welcome to *The New Rules of Pregnancy*. The mission of this book is to guide and support you with medical expertise while your body does what it knows how to do. Which is be pregnant. As doctors who have been enthusiastically caring for women for a couple of decades, we know that pregnancy is a robust process; the job is to keep the body safe and let it be. One of our goals is to take anxiety out of the equation and restore some of the glow to pregnancy. In our work, we've often wished there were a positive, concise guide, containing the most important information, that we could give to our pregnant patients. Something clear and uncluttered that reflected our compassionate, demedicalized, natural approach and cultivated a sense of well-being. We couldn't find that book, so we wrote it. *The New Rules of Pregnancy* explains everything you can do on the outside to support what's happening inside your body—and guides you through labor, delivery, and the beginning of motherhood. Our advice is frank and actionable—we get straight to the point, with evidence-based medicine that cuts a clear path. The idea is to help you take care of the things you can control and not make yourself crazy about those you can't—to encourage you to prepare for what's ahead but also have faith in the process. One of the best things you can do for your pregnancy is relax. By bringing you the tools we feel you really need in a spirit of calm and joy, we hope we can help you do that.

———

For starters, we want to encourage you to look forward. Dreaming about the birth of your baby—even at the beginning of pregnancy—helps you figure out what you want. And thinking even further ahead to postpartum healing and life as parents can help you and your partner prepare for the phases you'll go through together. Some people are really surprised (even shocked) by the life changes that come with pregnancy and recovery, but there's no reason you need to be. Just keep talking and anticipating what's next, staying on the same team. The adjustments we recommend in this book aren't necessarily difficult, but they're important. We're going to encourage you to slow down, to eat well, and in general to lean in to pregnancy. There's no such thing as a perfect pregnancy or a perfect birth, so don't pressure yourself to experience this process a certain way. Just take care—and take naps—and take your time where maybe you used to rush. For this particular 280-day stretch, your body is making a human. Go with that.

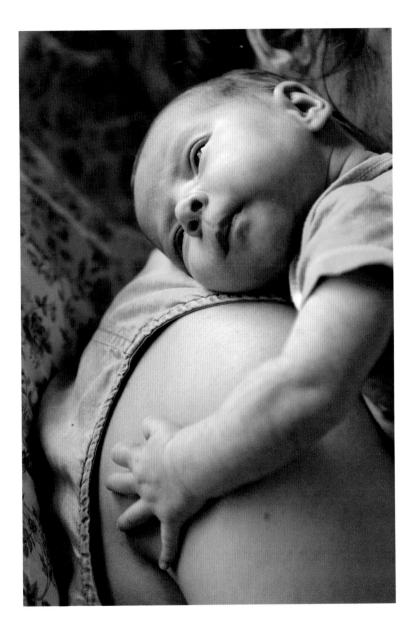

Eating & Drinking

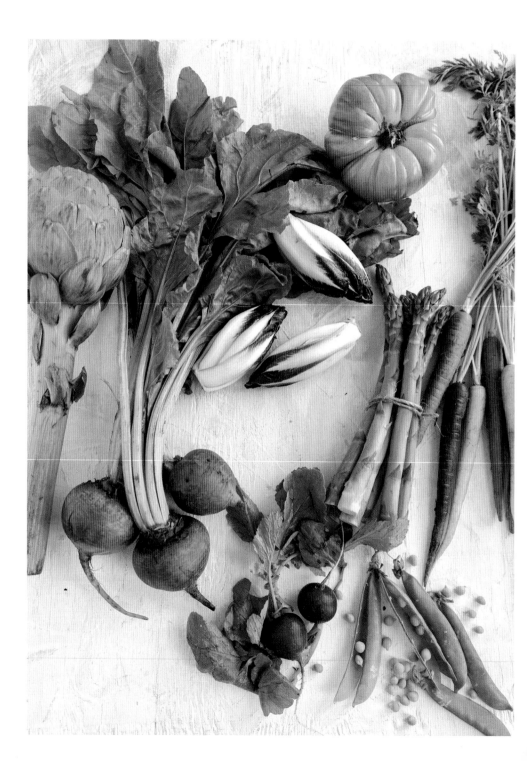

EAT CLEAN

Pregnancy offers a natural reset for health habits. Enjoy the opportunity, keep things simple, and don't stress. It's not hard to nourish yourself and get all that your body needs. The key is to lean on nutrient-dense fresh foods that give you the most benefits per bite—organic, hormone-free, antibiotic-free. Do what you can to avoid processed stuff (not just snacks from the vending machine but anything packaged—fresh is best). If you have access to a farmers' market, take advantage—a rainbow assortment of vegetables and fruits is always a good thing. Cook meat and fish well. Take care where you buy prepared foods—stick with clean, reliable sources. Nutrition specs are on the next pages. You'll get a lot from your prenatal vitamin (see page 41), but it's only part of the story; nutrients from food are absorbed better, and eating well can also help you feel your best.

PROTEIN, CALCIUM, FIBER

Protein makes babies grow. You want to build your pregnancy diet around it and aim to get somewhere between 60 and 70 grams a day. For reference, a chicken cutlet has about 25 grams of protein; a cup of lentils has 18. Two eggs deliver about 12 grams, and a half cup of tempeh is 15. A serving of salmon or steak has a whopping 40 grams of protein. If you're vegan by preference, consider eating eggs (and add Bragg's nutritional yeast to soups, avocado toast, or smoothies). If you're on the fence about meat, now is a good time to opt in. Calcium—also essential in pregnancy—builds babies' bones and teeth. Get 1,000 milligrams a day (a yogurt has 300 milligrams). Fiber is important for you, not the baby—to keep your digestive system working well. Have 28 grams a day (a serving of broccoli has 5 grams; a cup of raspberries has 8). This plan not only keeps you nourished but also keeps you full, so you're less likely to reach for foods without benefits (you know: bagels, cupcakes). Don't worry too much about precision—the amounts here are just guidelines. If you like, you can do an occasional check with an app like MyFitnessPal. Just type in what you ate that day to see how it all breaks down in terms of nutrients, then tweak as needed.

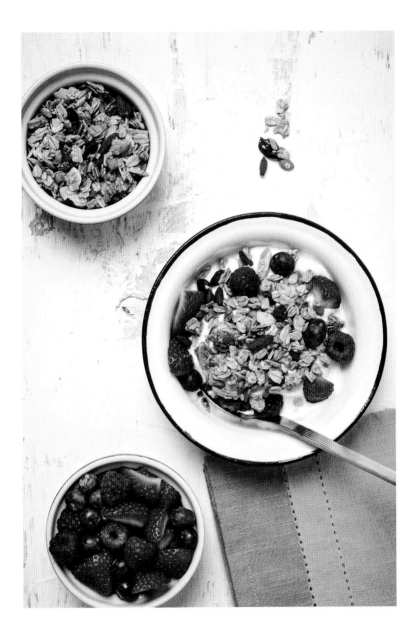

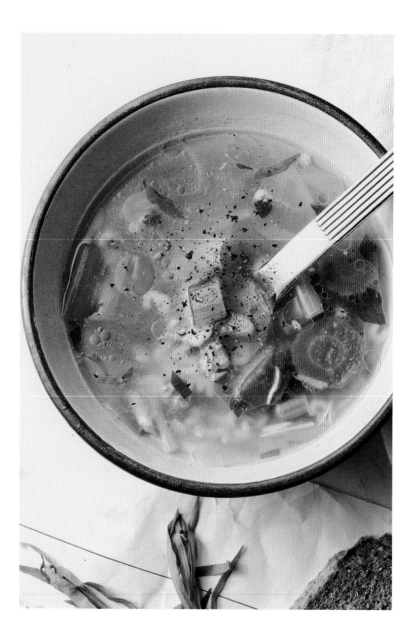

YOU'RE EATING FOR ONE

You only need to add about 400 calories a day to your diet, and those new calories should come from nutrient-dense foods. Wait till the second trimester to up your calories (if you start pregnancy underweight, your doctor might direct you to do it sooner). Think dairy, eggs, lean meat, dark leafy greens, cruciferous vegetables, and good fats like nuts and avocado. The omega-3 fatty acid DHA, which is found in fish, is especially important in pregnancy. You can get what you need by having two servings a week of low-mercury fish—sardines, salmon, trout, shrimp, pollack, canned light tuna (don't eat high-mercury fish: marlin, skate, shark, swordfish, tilefish, ahi tuna, king mackerel); if you're a vegetarian, you'll get your DHA from your prenatal vitamin. Ideal weight gain in pregnancy is not the same for everyone. Your doctor will tell you how much she'd like you to gain depending on your starting weight. For most people, it's somewhere between 25 and 35 pounds. If you keep an eye on portion size, fill up on protein and fiber, and don't overdo the carbs, the weight should work out. This is important. Gaining too much is not just about having more weight to lose on the other end; it also raises your risk for certain complications, including gestational diabetes.

SIX SMALL MEALS

Your digestive system is slowed by progesterone during pregnancy, and there's an uptick in gas. Eating smaller, more frequent meals is a great strategy. It's easier to digest less food in a sitting. Speaking of sitting, even if you're having a busy day, try to sit down when you eat; take your time and chew thoroughly. If needed, digestive aids Beano, Lactaid, Mylicon, and Tums are fine, but don't take more than the specified dose. Smaller meals can also help if you're experiencing nausea. An empty stomach is not great (you're more likely to feel nauseated when there's nothing in your stomach), so frequent light eating is a better bet. If you're coping with morning nausea, see if you can get down a small breakfast of carbs plus protein (an egg and half a piece of toast, say, or last night's chicken and rice). Fat can be hard to digest when you're nauseated, so hold off on foods like avocado and yogurt till later in the day. Acid reflux is another side effect of pregnancy hormones; avoid tomato sauce, mints, fried foods, carbonated drinks, and vinegar (enjoy olive oil, a healthy fat, on salad)—and don't lie down right after eating.

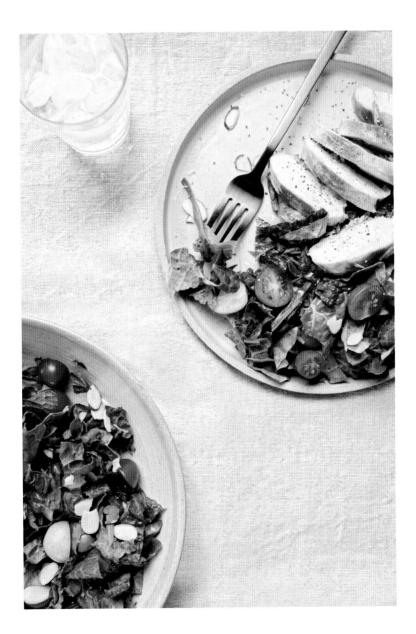

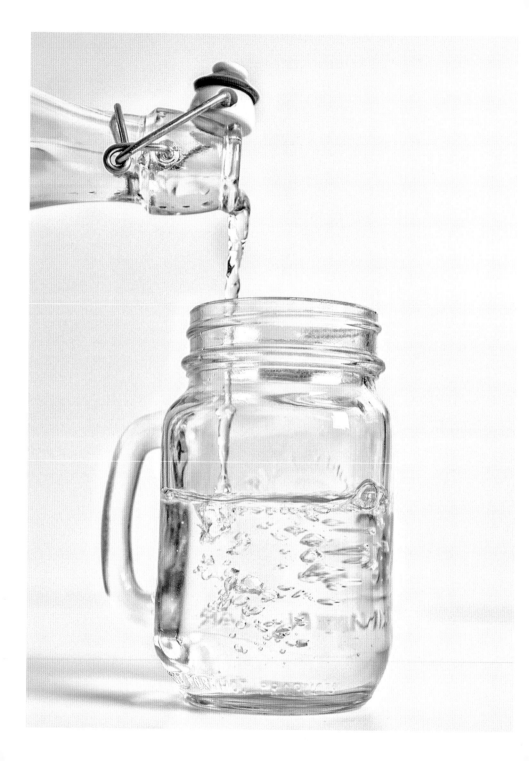

DRINK LOTS OF WATER

Filter your water and have about eight glasses a day. It helps your cardiovascular system, reduces constipation, and prevents UTIs. If you're not a fan of plain water, add mint or lemon (wash citrus skin if you're going to put it in your drink). Drinking plenty of water also lowers the risk of blood clots, which can be a serious issue during pregnancy (see page 57). Use a glass or a stainless-steel water bottle—the BPAs in some plastic bottles can be endocrine disruptors. If you're coping with nausea and vomiting and can barely keep anything down in the first trimester, don't worry too much about nutrients, but do stay focused on hydration—this is so important; you can also sip ice-cold sports drinks or Pedialyte to replace electrolytes. Otherwise, it's water, water everywhere and all the time, from the minute you know you're pregnant.

WASH PRODUCE WELL

Buy organic whenever possible, especially when it comes to fruits and vegetables eaten whole (without peeling)—things like apples and pears, berries and grapes, celery and spinach. Produce like avocados, citrus, melon, and corn, which has a protective outer layer that you'll discard, is hit less directly by pesticides. Throw away the outer leaves on conventionally grown lettuce, cabbage, and Brussels sprouts. Wash everything—organic or conventional—with a quick vinegar-water spritz. Water removes most pesticides, but vinegar addresses bacteria and mold spores. Mix one part distilled white vinegar and three parts water in a spray bottle; spritz produce, let sit for a minute, then rinse well with cold water. Or submerge fruits and veggies in a vinegar bath (same proportions—one part vinegar, three parts water), then rinse well. If you're storing produce, as opposed to eating it right away, be sure to dry it thoroughly.

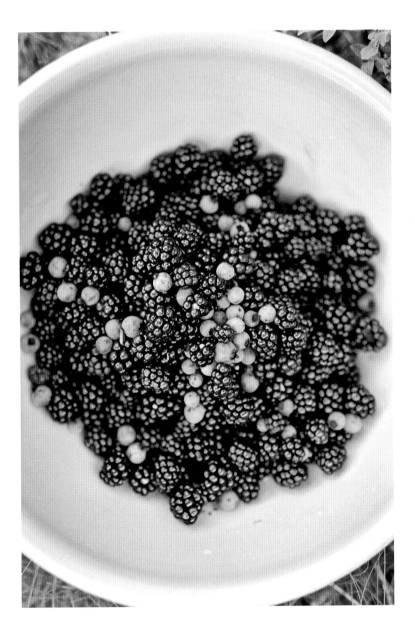

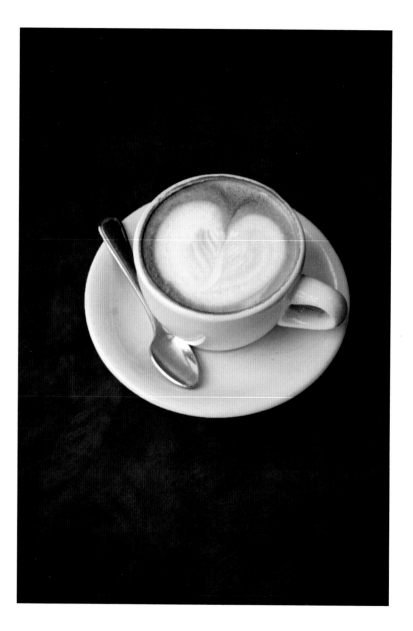

ONE GREAT CUP OF COFFEE

If you're inclined to drop caffeine while you're pregnant, you'll get no resistance here. Otherwise, keep consumption down to one cup of coffee per day. Make it count. Maybe you'll skip the morning coffee at home because the one you have at your desk (or after lunch) is more important to your mood or productivity. Black tea has about half the caffeine of coffee, so you can have two cups. Any combo that keeps you down to 200 milligrams of caffeine a day is fine. Enjoy caffeine-free teas like chamomile, mint, and ginger, but check the caffeine content of herbal blends. In general, approach herbal blends with caution (scientific studies haven't been done on all the ingredients they may contain). Or make your own blend, with decaf green or black tea plus fresh citrus rinds (wash them first) and cinnamon. So much coffee and tea drinking is about ritual, so if cutting back is tough, make a new ritual that comes with less (or no) caffeine—like taking a walk to refill your water bottle.

SAVE CERTAIN FOODS FOR LATER

Runny cheese, smoked fish, pâté, hollandaise sauce, steak tartare, raw fish—this is the feast you can have after you've stopped nursing. While you're pregnant and breastfeeding, stay away from these foods and others that could present a risk of listeria, salmonella, or other contaminants. Though the odds may be small, the impact on pregnancy can be serious. Stay away from raw or bloody meat, foods that might contain raw egg (certain mayos and salad dressings—check the label or ask the server), hot dogs, jerky, and deli meats. Bean sprouts and alfalfa sprouts are impossible to clean properly, which means they can harbor bacteria. Skip them. If you're traveling outside the United States, be mindful that some dairy products may not be pasteurized; in France, pregnant women are told not to eat salad greens and raw fruit and vegetables at restaurants, due to concerns about toxoplasmosis (it's more prevalent abroad). A lot of patients ask us about product recalls. Don't panic. If you've eaten something that's then been recalled and you have symptoms like fever and diarrhea, call your doctor. If you have no symptoms but are freaking out, you can still call your doctor. Basically, you can *always* call your doctor.

A TREAT A DAY

We advocate a low-sugar diet (because a no-sugar diet is going to stress you out). Aside from everything you probably already know about the havoc sugar can wreak on our bodies, studies link high sugar consumption in pregnant women to infant asthma and allergies, among other things. Say no to soda and candy—and to diet soda too; it's full of chemical sweeteners (which also cause gas). Keep artificial sweeteners out of your coffee, and skip gum (more sweeteners); you're better off using mouthwash. Fruit juice and dried fruit are intense concentrations of sugar; eat a whole piece of fruit instead (you'll benefit from the fiber). If you want to enjoy a small sweet once a day, pick something nutrient-dense like dark chocolate rather than a vending machine offering. Pair it with fiber (say, an apple), which slows absorption. This way your blood sugar won't spike, then crash.

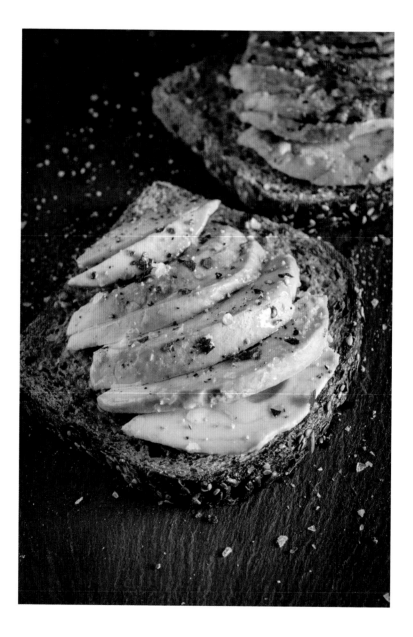

EXTRA EVERYTHING IF YOU'RE HAVING TWINS

Taking care of yourself while carrying twins means turning up the dial a little on everything that nourishes you. Extra rest, extra protein, extra folic acid, extra water. You should increase your caloric intake by 600 calories a day and take a prenatal vitamin with 1 milligram of folic acid. Recommended weight gain is about 10 pounds more when you're having twins, and doctor visits are more frequent; there's an increased chance of complications with twins, so you need extra care. Your doctor will guide you on exercise recommendations. Twins often mean a shorter pregnancy. They usually deliver earlier than the full nine months, and about half come before 37 weeks, in which case they may require extra time in the hospital.

CRAVINGS: MAGIC OR SCIENCE?

Both. With the increased blood flow of pregnancy comes turned-up senses—especially olfaction, which is entwined with the sense of taste. High estrogen (also part of pregnancy) affects the way your brain processes sensory information. Cravings and food aversions are all part of this sauce. Some women might experience a metallic or sour taste in the mouth in the first trimester (it's called dysgeusia, and while it can be annoying, it's not dangerous). A craving for acidic food can be a response to this, hence the urge for pickles. But some cravings are just messages from your body: You crave meat when you're lacking iron. (Another sign of iron deficiency, believe it or not, is an urge to chew ice.) Have some meat (or beans, if you're a vegetarian). There's no way to control this stuff short of a sensory deprivation tank. Just ride the wave and keep your sense of humor.

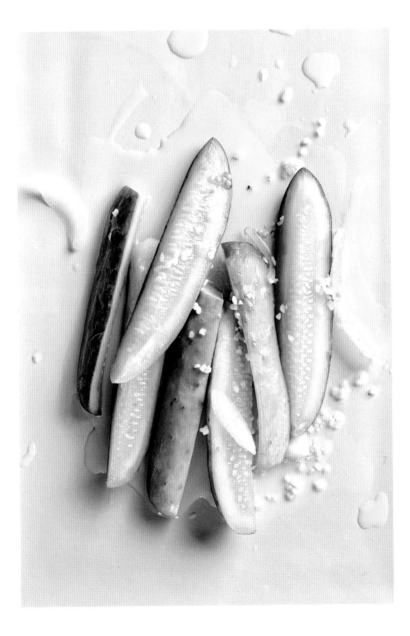

Everyday
Life

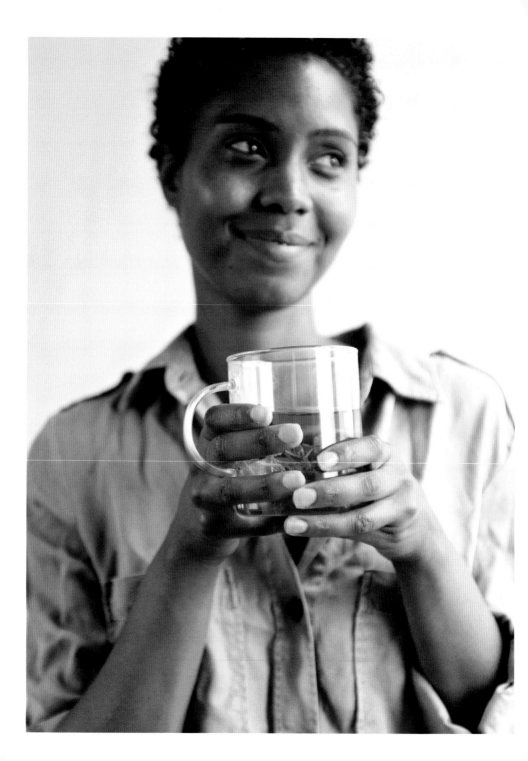

SLOW DOWN

Some stresses in life are unavoidable, and some we can control. When possible during pregnancy, take the opportunity to ease up. Reevaluate your schedule and prioritize rest—even if you have a high-tempo personality and lifestyle. Normal everyday stress shouldn't adversely affect the baby, but rushing around at warp speed is not great (it floods your body with cortisol and also can put you at risk for a fall). Look for small and large ways to lighten your load. Go to bed earlier, and leave yourself extra time in the morning to get ready for work. Dress comfortably, and don't worry about whether you're "pregnant enough" for maternity clothes (the first time you step into a pair of maternity jeans, the relief can be palpable). Skip that event you didn't really want to go to. Catch the next train instead of hustling for the one about to pull in. Hold the banister. Accept that seat someone kindly offers. This is a special (and finite) time. Take it easy.

SOAP AND WATER,
ALL DAY LONG

Protecting yourself against germs is a priority during pregnancy, and plain old handwashing goes a long way. Hot water isn't even required; cold works just as well. What *does* matter is that you don't rush through (wash for as long as it takes to sing a whole verse of a song). Clean between your fingers like a surgeon, rinse well, and don't use funky-seeming shared hand towels. Opt for regular soap over antibacterial—and actual soap and water over antiseptic sanitizers. In a pinch, using a sanitizer is better than not cleansing germy hands, but the safety of additives in some of these products is still being investigated, so don't make a habit of it. Wash up more frequently than you're used to—especially after hanging out with kids, riding public transportation, and using shared equipment, like a supermarket cart. Check labels, and don't buy soaps or sanitizers (or anything, for that matter) containing triclosan, which is a potential hormone disruptor.

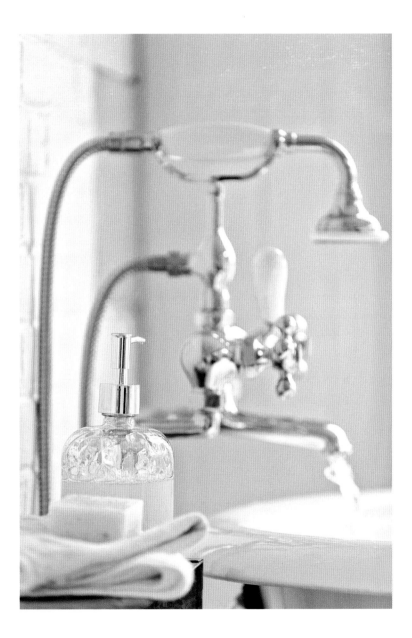

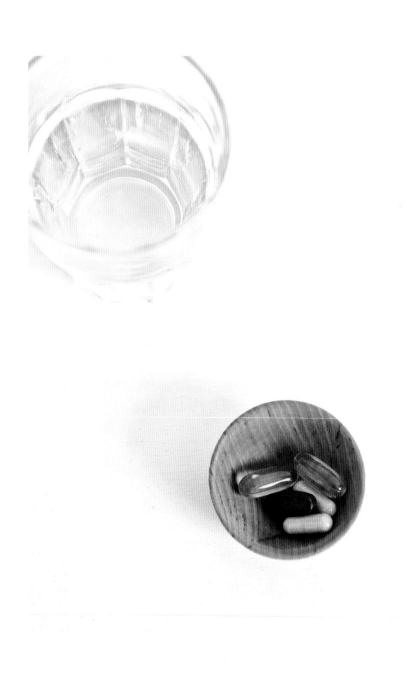

YOUR PRENATAL VITAMIN

Take a vitamin with at least 600 micrograms of folic acid (some people can't absorb certain forms of folate, so we recommend the methylated form, which is fine for all) and 300 milligrams of DHA. If you're reading this book in advance of becoming pregnant, feel free to start taking a prenatal vitamin now. You also need at least 27 milligrams of iron every day. If you eat beef, you can depend on your diet for some of this (a serving of steak has about 6 milligrams of iron; a burger has about 2). One of the reasons meat, fish, and poultry are so beneficial is that the form of iron they deliver is more easily absorbed than the iron that comes from legumes or vegetables. So if you don't eat meat, be sure your vitamin has at least 27 milligrams of iron. Vitamin C increases iron absorption, so add citrus to iron-rich foods (fresh lemon dressing on your spinach salad, for example). Remember, iron can cause constipation—which plenty of fiber, water, and exercise will mitigate.

COMBATING NAUSEA

If you're finding it difficult to eat, nibble on low-salt crackers or anything else you can tolerate. Don't let your stomach become too empty or too full. Ask your doctors about temporarily switching to a prenatal vitamin without iron (iron can contribute to nausea). Nausea is often rooted in the sense of smell, so sniffing things like peppermint can help. More ideas:

- Apply peppermint lip balm when you wake up, or use peppermint or lemongrass roll-on on your wrists.

- Take vitamin B_6 (25 milligrams every eight hours).

- Apply pressure to the inside of your wrist (a pressure point known as P-6). Press with the opposite thumb, or wear a slip-on elastic wristband marketed for seasickness or pregnancy.

- Suck on anti-nausea candies like Preggie Pop Drops.

- Try a BRAT diet (bananas, rice, applesauce, toast). Add plain chicken if and when you can.

- Exercise, even though it may be the last thing you feel like doing when you're queasy. Some women find it helps with nausea.

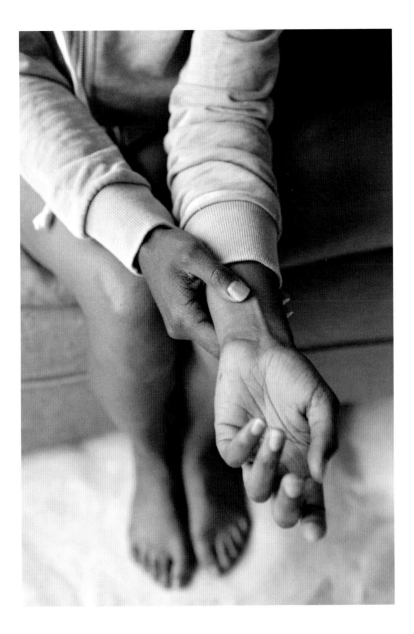

IF THE NAUSEA
DOESN'T STOP

For most women who experience nausea and exhaustion in the first trimester, relief comes by week 13 or 14. Hormones change, and the discomfort lifts. Energy ramps up, and you start to feel like yourself again. But there's a percentage of women for whom pregnancy is one long physical trial; they don't get that relief at 13 weeks and instead feel weary and unwell for the whole nine months. If you're having this experience, we know it's rough—especially if you've seen friends breeze through with rosy cheeks and a smile. It can be especially frustrating if you've been looking forward to pregnancy as a high point of life. It's normal to be a little resentful or to feel like something's been stolen from you—the gift of a comfortable pregnancy. We're not going to try to negate those feelings. The only solace we can offer is that you're not alone in feeling this way, and eventually these 40 weeks will pass.

MIXED FEELINGS
ARE NORMAL

There's a lot of cultural pressure to be happy when you're pregnant. But not everyone feels this way. Ambivalence is really common. Bringing new life into the world pushes all the big philosophical buttons. It can be jarring. A bit of anxiety about the impending life changes is not necessarily something to worry about. And if you don't particularly like being pregnant, that's okay too. Don't get hung up on it. It doesn't mean you won't be a great mother. But if you feel completely overwhelmed or are dealing with despair, please seek help. Struggling in pregnancy might be a marker for postpartum depression, so you want to have a therapist in place, stay connected to friends, and talk openly with your partner and your caregiver.

MOVE AROUND AT WORK

You want to avoid stasis in pregnancy, even down to switching which leg is crossed on top now and then. Since a lot of us spend eight hours a day sitting at work, that's a time to be aware. Get up every twenty minutes if possible and stretch or take a walk, inside or out (set your phone to ding as a prompt, to train yourself). Do an in-house errand. Take the long route to the printer. Go have a face-to-face chat instead of sending an email. Anything that moves your limbs and gets your circulation going. Also, make sure your workstation is set up for maximum comfort, so you're not hunching forward or tensing certain muscles all day long. Be sure your computer monitor and office chair are at ergonomically correct heights (your thighs should be parallel to the floor, with feet resting flat). Prop a lumbar pillow behind your back, or beneath your bum. Readjust for comfort as the baby grows and your body changes.

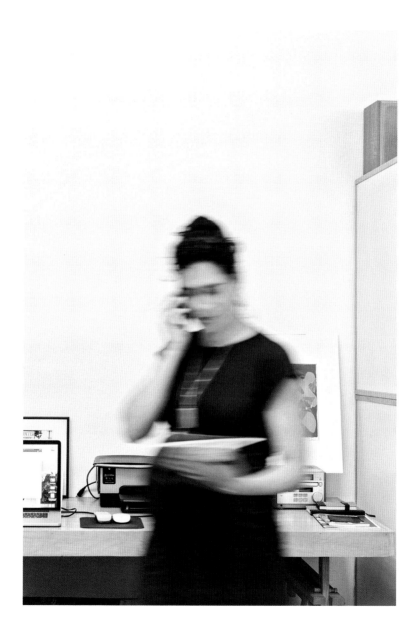

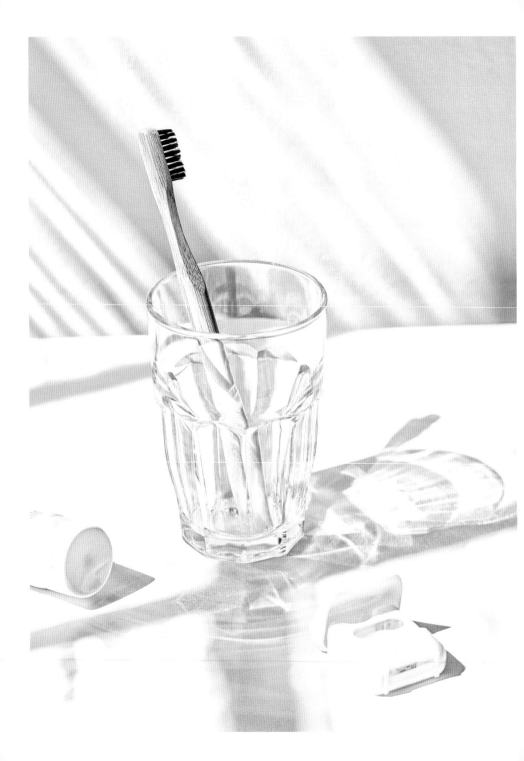

FLOSS EVERY DAY

Pregnancy hormones can increase your risk of gum issues like gingivitis. Gums may also have more of a tendency to become engorged and then to bleed. If you need dental work but it can wait, have it done in the second trimester (also the best time for a cleaning). Day to day, floss gently and regularly, brush with a toothpaste that doesn't contain triclosan (like Tom's of Maine), and use mouthwash (also triclosan-free). Sometimes gums can develop little benign growths during pregnancy—probably nothing to worry about, but tell your doctor if you notice anything. Hold off on teeth-whitening; you want to minimize exposure to chemicals. If you're reading this book prior to becoming pregnant, have your teeth checked now to avoid having to do major dental work while pregnant.

BREATHE FRESH AIR

Use common sense when it comes to indoor and outdoor toxins. Switch to nontoxic, bleach-free cleaning products and detergents, and wear gloves while cleaning. Rinse out filters on air conditioners and keep humidifiers and dehumidifiers wiped down to minimize any chance of mold (you can clean them with white vinegar). If the exterminator comes to spray for bugs, leave the house; open windows and wash anything that might have been exposed. Don't spend too much time in environments where chemicals are in heavy use. Choose nail salons that are clean and well ventilated (or do your nails at home). Skip projects that involve harsh glues or paints. At home, let in fresh air. Step outside of closed environments whenever you can, and fill your lungs. And give the kitchen a check. You want to use healthy materials when cooking, like enamel, stainless steel, and cast iron. Get rid of pans with coated surfaces that could peel (this advice isn't just for pregnancy). When storing ingredients or leftovers, opt for glass—some plastics can leach chemicals into food. If you're a vintage fan, watch out for glazed kitchenware. Some of that old-timey charm comes with lead in the glaze—it's fine to have around for decoration, but it's not necessarily safe for food.

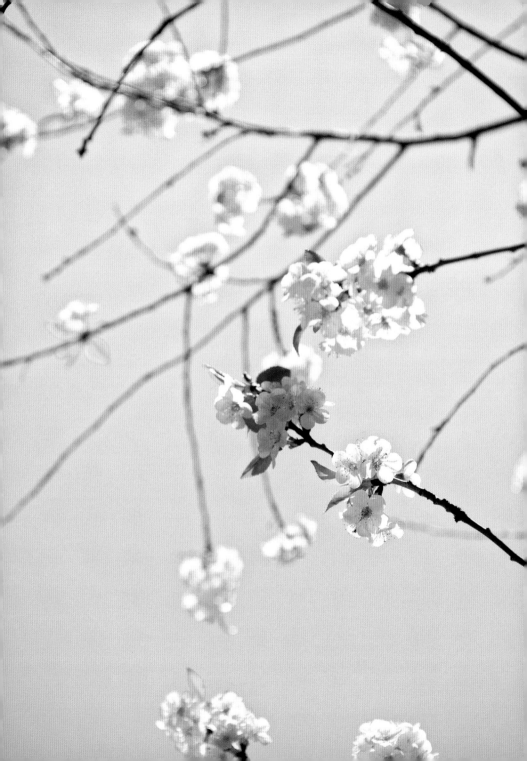

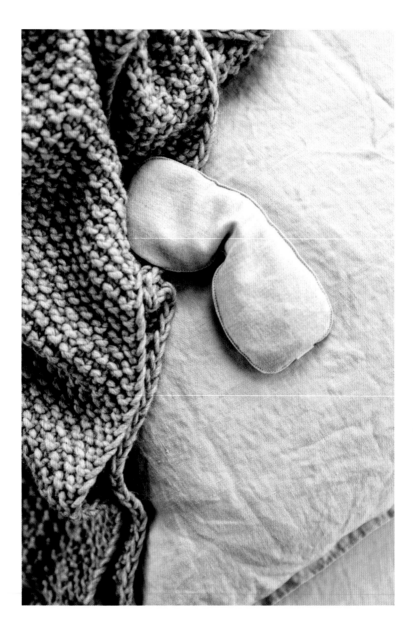

NATURAL SELF-CARE

Some medications are safe during pregnancy, but try to fix what ails you without medication when you can. If you have a headache, drink a big glass of water, use a cold compress, or rest with an eye pillow. For back pain, do some stretches (see page 121 for a yoga pose that addresses lower back pain), change your shoes, take a walk or a bath, or use a heating pad. If you feel generally crummy, take a day off and just sleep. Congestion is common in pregnancy; due to increased blood flow and mucus production, plus swollen membranes, you might feel perpetually stuffy. A dab of Vicks VapoRub under the nose can help. So can saline nose drops, a humidifier, and anti-snore strips. Some people find that acupuncture improves just about anything mentioned above. If on occasion you need to take an approved pain reliever (like Tylenol), cold medicine (like Mucinex), sleep aid (like Unisom), or any other approved over-the-counter medication, take it as briefly as possible, and in no more than the recommended dosage.

CHECK YOUR BEAUTY PRODUCTS

Anything you put on your skin can seep into your bloodstream, so look at labels. Avoid retinoids, hydroquinone, ammonia, phthalates, dihydroxyacetone, thioglycolic acid, propylene glycol, and BHT (butylated hydroxytoluene). Or just opt for something you know is chemical-free—especially when it comes to products that cover a lot of surface area, like the moisturizer you use from head to toe (think organic coconut oil, shea butter, or lotions from manufacturers like Weleda or Dr. Hauschka). Choose nail polish that's lighter on the chemicals: Ella & Mila, Tenoverten, and Nars are brands whose polishes are made without toluene, formaldehyde, and DBP (dibutyl phthalate). There's no evidence that hair dye is harmful during pregnancy, but there's also no evidence that it's safe. When you're aiming to minimize your exposure to toxins, it makes sense to take a break from chemical hair color and keratin. Consider using a plant-based product like henna, or go natural. If you're very worried about chemicals or simply want to know more, you can subscribe (for a fee) to the database Reprotox.org, a reliable source where you can look up specific ingredients. Please don't rely on random searches for information—stick with trusted, legit, well-researched sources.

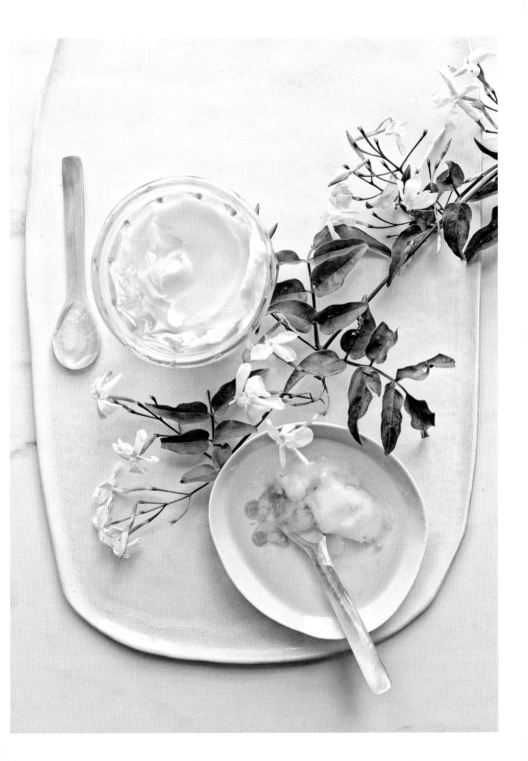

PREGNANCY SKIN

Pigmentation can be stimulated by pregnancy, so certain parts of your body may darken (like the linea nigra—that stripe from the navel down your lower belly). You might get patchy areas on your face, called melasma (also known by the overly dramatic name "the mask of pregnancy"). They usually fade within a year, but the sun can make them worse, so protect yourself. We want you to enjoy sunshine—it's great for your mood—but a sunburn is dehydrating, which is not safe. Wear a hat and use a zinc-oxide sunscreen rather than a chemical-based product (steer clear of the ingredient oxybenzone, which may not be safe in pregnancy). Avoid oily formulations, because you're already more prone to acne when you're pregnant (you can treat it with topical erythromycin gel or benzoyl peroxide). Pregnancy hormones can also sensitize skin, so don't use scrubs or get laser treatments, and forget Botox for now. It's not that these treatments are dangerous; it's just that they can irritate pregnant skin.

ABOUT BLOOD CLOTS

Pregnancy is a "hypercoagulable state," which just means it comes with an elevated risk of blood clots. Blood clots are dangerous and have the potential to be fatal. In pregnancy, they tend to form in the legs. Much of the general advice on taking care of yourself while pregnant protects you from blood clots: Drink plenty of water, stay active, don't sit still for long stretches or leave your legs in one position for extended periods—and take special care on airplanes (more about this on page 140). Some specific pregnancy factors that increase your risk of clots include obesity, twin pregnancy, diabetes, and varicose veins. If you're experiencing calf pain or swelling, stop whatever you're doing and call the doctor. In the first week postpartum, the risk of blood clots actually peaks and continues for six to eight weeks. This is one of the reasons it's so important to walk very early postpartum, whether you've had a Cesarean birth or a vaginal delivery.

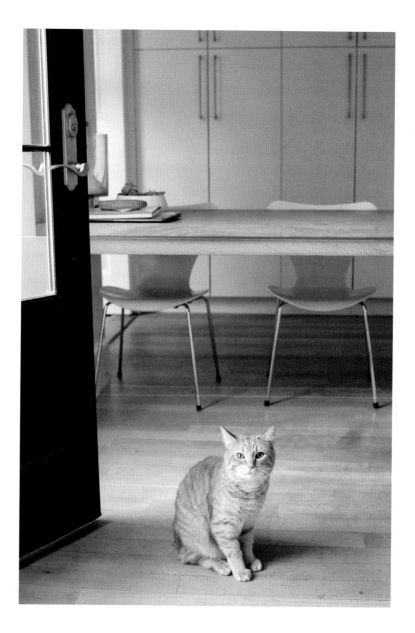

LOVE YOUR CAT,
BUT AVOID THE LITTER BOX

If you're a cat parent, you may have heard about toxoplasmosis, an infection cats can transmit—and one you need to avoid. It takes a fecal-oral route, meaning if your hand has been in contact with contaminated cat poop and that hand touches your mouth, you're at risk. Odds are this won't happen, but odds are better when you're not cleaning the litter box. So that job goes to your partner for now. If your cat never goes outside, then your home shouldn't be at risk because the true source of toxoplasmosis is raw meat (the mouse an outdoor cat catches and eats). But best to be cautious. In related news, ask your partner to take care of applying flea and tick drops, and let the medication soak in for a while before you cuddle with your pet.

STRETCH MARKS HAPPEN

. . . because the tissue under the skin grows faster than the skin can accommodate. They can occur during any trimester but are most common in the third. There's nothing that's been proven to prevent stretch marks, but there are a few things that might help: Shield vulnerable body parts—belly, breasts, thighs—from the sun while pregnant. Keep skin pliable with natural oils and lotions (coconut oil, olive oil, vitamin E cream, or blends like Kiehl's Mom & Baby Nurturing Body Oil), which can also relieve itching as your belly grows. Stay hydrated. Most likely, people develop stretch marks due to a genetic propensity, but the best chance of minimizing them comes back to the same advice you're probably already sick of hearing: Avoid extra weight gain.

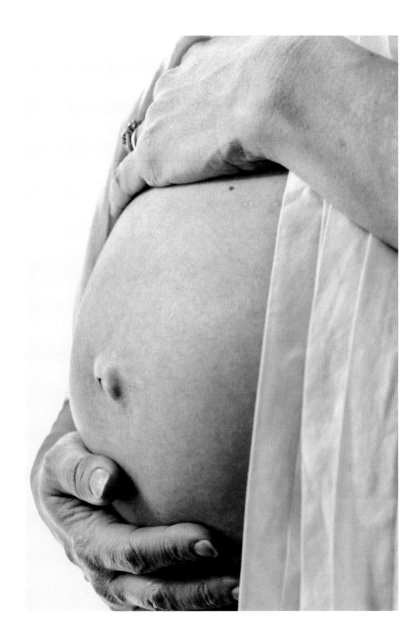

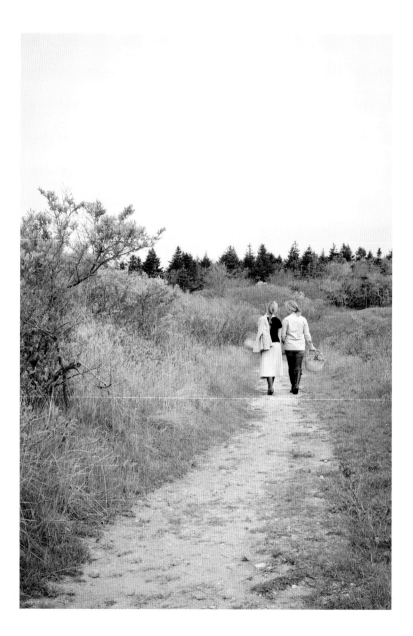

ENJOY NATURE

Time outside and gentle uphill hikes are fantastic for you, but wear long pants tucked into socks and tops with long fitted sleeves or jackets with elastic around the wrist. Light-colored clothing makes it easier to spot a tick when you check afterward (ask your partner or a friend for help—it's important). Same rules apply for the clothes you wear while gardening—just add gloves. Don't freak out if you find a tick on your skin—it takes twenty-four to thirty-six hours to transmit disease in most cases—but do call your doctor. Save the tick on a piece of Scotch tape for reference. If you want to, you can identify its type using the site TickEncounter.org.

HAVE SEX

. . . as often as you want, as long as your doctor doesn't say otherwise. Desire might come and go. In the first trimester, when you're feeling exhausted, and possibly nauseated, you may not be in the mood, but don't worry. That's not a sign of how you'll feel throughout pregnancy. Libido tends to get a boost in the second trimester as blood flow and hormones ramp up (and vaginal secretions increase). At any stage, though, if you're not into sex, talk with your partner rather than quietly retreating. Work through everything together. Communicating openly lets you enjoy other types of intimacy—holding hands, swapping neck massages—with less pressure. (And speaking of pressure, let us put your mind at ease if you're concerned: The penis is not hitting the baby or poking at the amniotic sac.) In the third trimester, you may have some difficulty with orgasm (it'll come back). And after 36 weeks, you might experience contractions after orgasm or see a bit of pink-stained mucus after intercourse. That's all right. As long as your doctor says it's okay, you can keep having sex. Lastly, some sex don'ts: no blowing into the vagina; no anal to vaginal sex; no lube with parabens, flavors, or warming activity; and no foreign objects inside. (Did we kill the mood?)

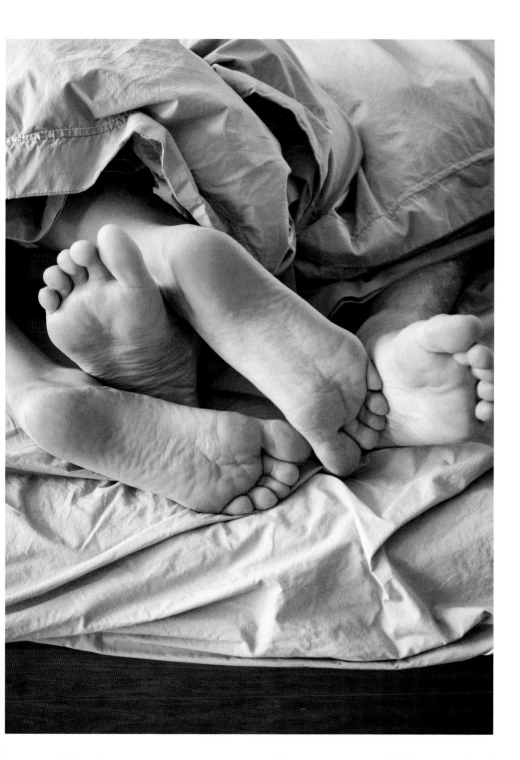

Thinking & Planning

TAKE YOUR TIME

Consider waiting till the first trimester passes and the risk of miscarriage drops significantly to go public with your pregnancy. Once you get to the second trimester, the chance of loss is quite low. Though it might be difficult to make it all the way to the 12-week mark with only your very closest in the know, it can also be a sweet time for you and your partner, while the secret is small. If something should go wrong, the fewer people you've told, the fewer you have to update. As your pregnancy progresses, don't feel pressured to report on every aspect of it. If you're a quiet type who'd rather not recount details of doctor visits, weight gain, and testing, that's okay. Maybe you want to add a week to your "public" due date to create a cushion of privacy, so you're not getting constant calls. Love comes in many forms, and that might include texts from your aunt about a listeria outbreak in a grocery store eighty miles from where you live. You don't necessarily have to engage. Be kind, but create the right boundaries for yourself, and don't feel guilty about it.

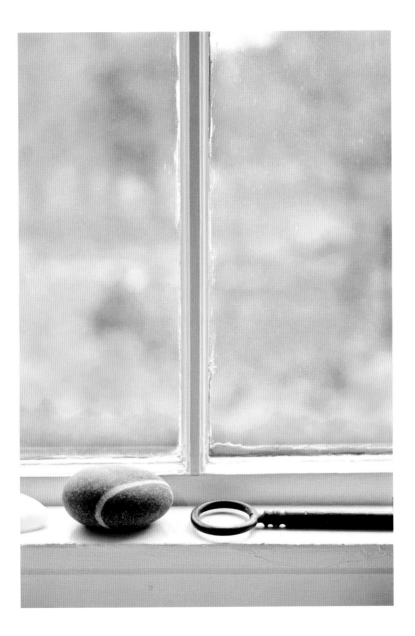

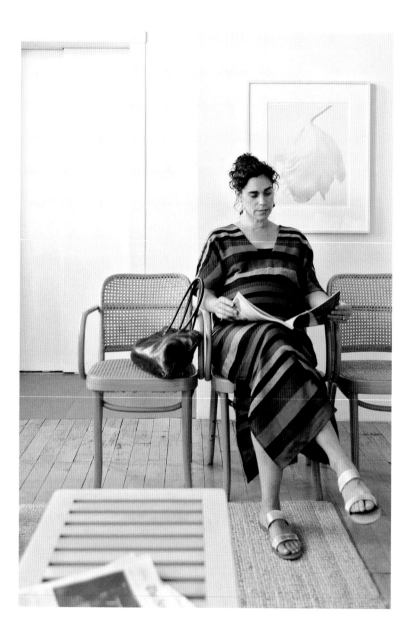

GETTING COMFORTABLE WITH YOUR CAREGIVERS

Most OBs run in packs. When you choose a doctor (somewhere at the intersection of philosophy, insurance, reputation, experience, location, availability, and affiliation with a good hospital), there's a good chance you'll end up with a large group. Typically with large practices, any of the doctors in that group (or midwives, if the practice includes midwives) could end up delivering your baby. You may be able to decide whether you want to see one doctor (*your* doctor) for all appointments, or meet other doctors in the practice over the course of your pregnancy—rotating your visits through the roster—so you're less likely to have an unfamiliar face taking you over the finish line. There are some small practices and solo OBs out there. If this is available to you, look into it; it may offer a more intimate experience. If you have any reason to expect a more complicated pregnancy (like you're having twins), this should inform your choice of caregiver: Pick a doctor at the hospital with the best NICU (neonatal intensive care unit) in your area.

WHEN CONSIDERING
A MIDWIFE

Midwifery practices are supportive of natural birth and tend to be less rushed and more relaxed than medical practices are able to be. But a midwife's scope of practice is normal pregnancy. So if you choose a midwife, be sure you understand what the plan is if things don't go routinely. If your pregnancy or delivery becomes complicated, you'll need a doctor to step in and either collaborate with your midwife or fully take over your care. A great midwife has great backup. Learn about the backup doctor as if she's your actual health-care provider. It should be someone with a lot of experience, with a good reputation, who has done a lot of births and has good backup herself. Use all the same tools you'd use in evaluating any caregiver, including consideration of the birthing center or hospital where your midwife and backup doctor deliver. One specific reason some people opt for midwives is that they want a home birth. We understand the appeal of home birth, but we don't recommend it in the United States. We want you in a setting where medical resources are readily available, just in case. A hospital is a building full of safety tools. It's the place with all the stuff and expertise needed if things don't go as planned.

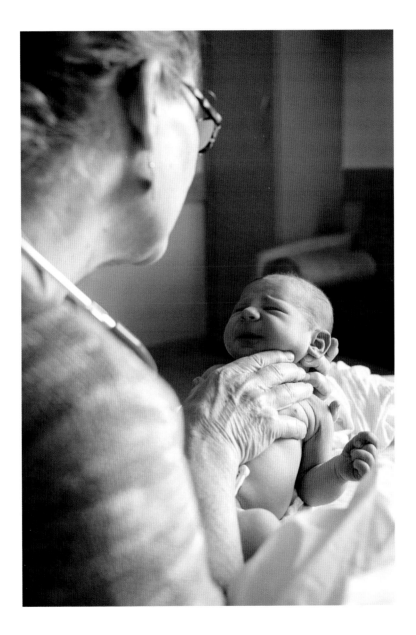

THE CASE FOR A LABOR DOULA

Most hospitals allow one person (your partner) plus a support person in the room—that would be a labor doula, a trained, experienced person providing continuous support for the laboring mother. We've seen great results with labor doulas. Patients have told us that doulas have helped them feel empowered, strong, safe, and clear during labor. If you're interested, ask early if your caregiver works with doulas. Some doctors and midwives don't. There are caregivers who feel a doula interferes with the relationship between partners. We've found the opposite to be true. Birth is hard work, and there's no nice neat, civilized way to do it. The responsibility given to partners in the birth experience is a little outsize. They can get scared. In the moment, they may not know what to do—why should they? A doula makes everyone feel calmer and more in control—she normalizes the situation. Our patients and their partners—*especially* their partners—have without exception been really happy they made the decision to go with a doula. Also, doulas tend to decrease the chance of interventions that can lead to a Cesarean birth. Some people ask, *Why a doula and not a family member?* The essential feature of a doula is that she's seen a lot of births.

Usually that's not true of a family member. And the emotional distance a doula has can be beneficial. If it's something that fits in your budget, please consider a doula. Fees vary based on region, number of births, and a few other factors. A personal recommendation is a great way to find the right person (begin your search at around 20 weeks), but another starting point is a doula certifying organization such as DONA International (DONA.org). Meet, chat, check references.

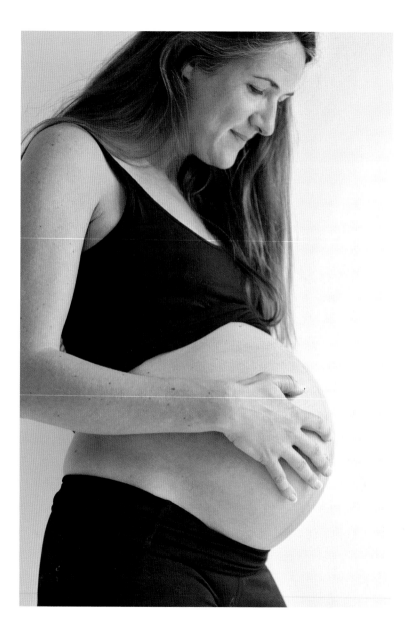

ABOUT PAIN RELIEF IN LABOR

Some patients talk to us about unspoken (and spoken) pressure to have an unmedicated birth. We understand. While it's wonderful if you *want* to try for an unmedicated birth, we all have different circumstances. Some labors are longer than others. Some of us have different pain thresholds. So many factors come together that might make an unmedicated birth possible in some situations and not others. This is your unique birth—a private matter for you, your partner, and your baby. If you want a natural birth, go for it. Put your best team and strategy together and focus your efforts on it. Go as far as you can, but keep an open mind. The length of your labor might change things. The time course is not something we can predict. If ultimately you need a little help or even a *lot* of help toward the end, embrace the fact that you gave it your best shot and that we live in a time when options are available. In our experience, this approach—taking yourself as far as you can and then using science and medicine to help you finish—leads to high personal satisfaction. It doesn't have to be an all-or-nothing mentality. An "almost unmedicated birth" can be extremely gratifying. We also have patients who know ahead of time that they want nothing to do with an unmedicated birth. "Epidural, please," they say as soon as they get to the hospital. If you want pain medicine right away, it's your right to have it. Be clear and ask your doctor, and she will help you. Most of all, give yourself some leeway. It may be impossible to predict how you're going to feel and what you're going to need, and that's okay. You don't have to know in advance.

MEDICATIONS COMMONLY USED WITH BIRTH

Pitocin is an IV medication that increases the strength and frequency of contractions. It's used to help labor advance, or sometimes to start labor. After delivery, most likely you'll be given a little Pitocin to help the uterus contract and reduce the chance of postpartum hemorrhage (heavy bleeding after delivery).

Epidural anesthesia—referred to simply as an epidural—is the most common pain medication for labor. At some hospitals, an epidural is used in more than 90 percent of births. The medicine is delivered through a very thin tube inserted in the lower back. An epidural usually eliminates all the pain, but it can also make you numb from the waist down. Because it affects the muscle strength in your lower body, an epidural changes your labor from one where you can be upright with your feet on the ground to one where you're lying in bed. This means you no longer have gravity working with you. That said, for a low-pain birth, there's nothing like it. If you're scheduled for a Cesarean, you'll get something similar—a single-shot spinal anesthesia that lasts two to three hours.

Nitrous oxide, also known as "gas and air," is the same stuff the dentist uses and is administered the same way—you just hold a mask up to your face and breathe. It can be used on the way to the epidural or potentially as an alternative to an epidural. Nitrous oxide doesn't make the pain go away, but as some people say, it makes you care less about it—and this can be especially helpful at the end of labor. It's short-acting; if you don't like the way it feels, it can be out of your system quickly. Ask your doctor in advance if it's available to you—it's not in all hospitals yet, but its popularity is growing.

PERSPECTIVE ON
A CESAREAN BIRTH

A C-section doesn't erase all your other wishes for the birth experience. You can still have a lot of the elements of a vaginal birth. In fact, there's something going on at Brigham and Women's Hospital, affiliated with Harvard, that's informally referred to as a "gentle C-section"; it offers a wonderful template for a great Cesarean birth experience, and many of the details are reasonable requests to include in a birth plan (you definitely want to include your wishes related to a Cesarean, in case it should happen). Some are simple adjustments that can set up a new mother having a Cesarean to more easily hold and nurse the baby immediately after delivery (for example, the anesthesiologist can put the EKG leads on the mother's back instead of on her chest so the wires won't be in the way of skin-to-skin bonding with the newborn; the pulse monitor that measures her heart rate and oxygen status can be clipped to an ear instead of a finger, freeing up her hand). In our birth plan suggestions on page 152, you'll see these ideas, plus others. If you'd like to learn more about gentle C's, search "Brigham gentle C-section" online.

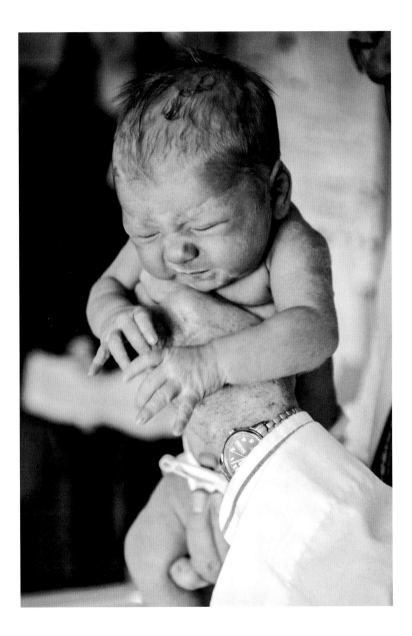

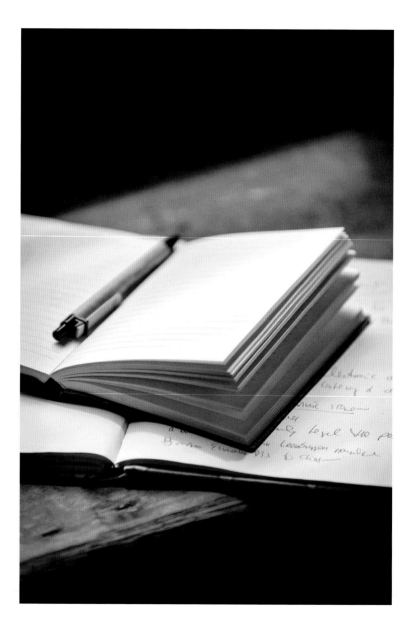

THINK OF A BIRTH PLAN
AS A WISH LIST

Writing a birth plan can give you a sense of ownership over the process. But while some caregivers love birth plans, there are others who don't—and the longer the plan, the more it can raise hackles. The medical team helping you through labor and delivery has one goal: healthy baby and healthy mother. Nothing else comes close to this in importance. This doesn't mean the crew doesn't want you to have a great birth experience. It just means their energies and efforts are focused on the outcome, as they should be. That's why a birth plan is more of a wish list than anything else. If that mind-set can inform your approach, it will make all the difference. Go short (most people should be able to get everything they need on a single page). Be kind and polite. Don't get too medical (unless you're an OB)—focus more on the spirit of the birth than on the technical aspects. For suggestions on specifics to include in your birth plan, see page 152.

OBSESSING OVER
WHAT CAN GO WRONG

. . . doesn't make things go right. It only raises your blood pressure and stress hormone levels and keeps you awake at night. Try to stay off the internet when it comes to issues related to your pregnancy, especially if you know you're the worrying type. It's tempting to look up every twinge in search of assurance that nothing is wrong. But health info taken out of context is not necessarily helpful. Keep a list of questions on your phone and a pad on your nightstand. Just the act of writing things down is calming—getting the thoughts out of your head and onto paper (or screen—with a list app). You can fire off all these questions during your next doctor's appointment; if you have a pressing concern, call. And if you really need to look something up, stick with MayoClinic.org.

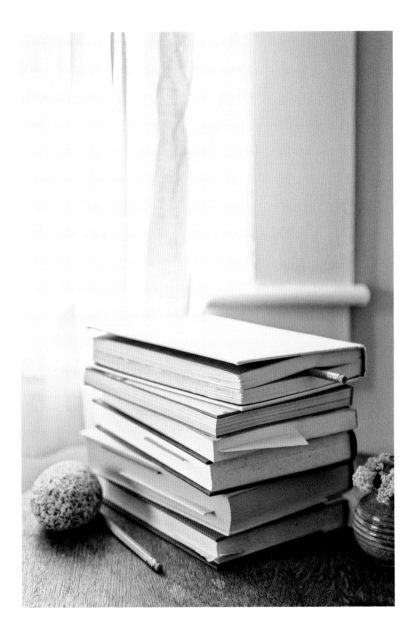

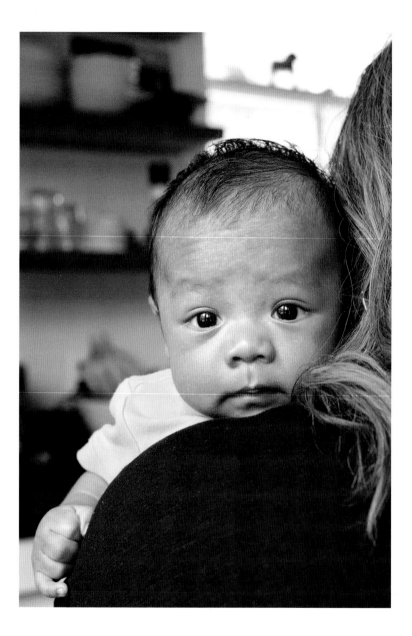

WHY NURSING MATTERS

You probably already know this, but we just want to re-iterate why breastfeeding is so healthy for both you and your baby, and why the American Academy of Pediatrics (AAP.org) recommends babies receive nothing but breast milk till six months, when it's time for solid foods. Breastfeeding transfers your antibodies to the baby and helps build his microbiome. It lowers his risk of allergies and asthma, and it may fortify him against obesity and cardiovascular disease. The baby's suck helps your uterus shrink back to normal size. Nursing decreases your risk of endometriosis and cancer. And it bonds you to your baby. All of this said, if there's some reason you can't nurse—there's a small percentage of women whose bodies just don't produce milk, as much as they try—or if breastfeeding has negative associations for you, it's not the end of the world. Let yourself off the hook, and don't feel bad about it.

WHAT IF I DON'T WANT
MY PARTNER TO WATCH?

If you'd prefer your partner not see the moment of birth, that's fine. There's more than one way to do this together. And the way your friend or your sister or your cousin did it may not be right for you. It's totally legitimate to feel uncomfortable at the notion of your partner watching you push out a baby—not that long ago, partners weren't even in the delivery room. On points like this that are not a matter of safety, talk it through. Make a plan. Have it your way. This is your unique birth. We would like to open the door to the idea that you don't have to share parts of it if you don't want to.

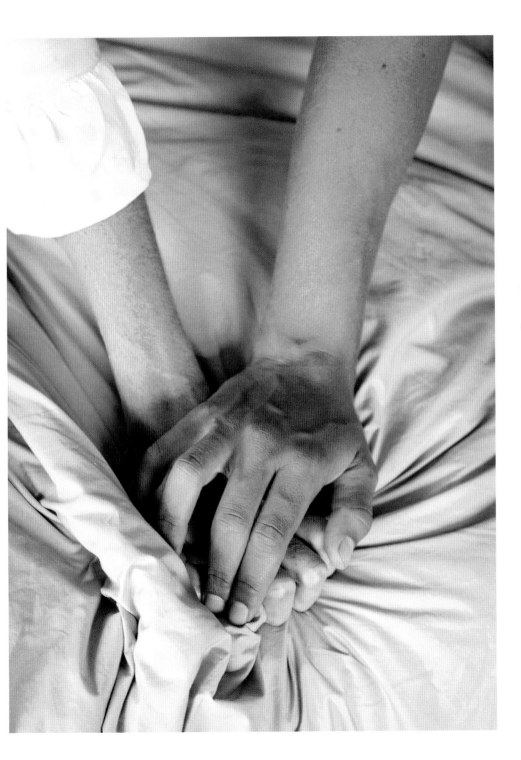

Seeing Your Doctor

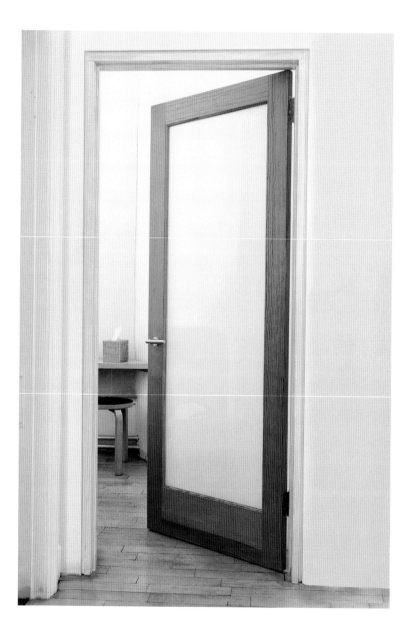

YOUR FIRST APPOINTMENT

With a typical pregnancy, you'll see your caregiver once a month for the first six months, then every two weeks beginning around week 28. After 36 weeks, appointments might be weekly. At your first prenatal visit, your provider will likely give you a due date based on your last menstrual period or an early sonogram. You'll get a physical exam (blood pressure, weight, and breast/pelvic exam with a Pap smear, if you're due for one). You'll answer lots of questions about your medical history. Your blood type and Rh status and immunity to certain viruses like chicken pox and rubella will be checked. You'll be tested for infections (including STIs) that require treatment so the baby is protected in utero and at birth. You'll learn about screenings for genetic conditions like cystic fibrosis, sickle cell disease, spinal muscular atrophy, and fragile X syndrome (if you're reading this book in advance of becoming pregnant, you can have these screenings done now). Your blood count (and maybe thyroid levels) will also be checked.

TESTS IN PREGNANCY

Some prenatal visits will be quick—weight and blood pressure, a urine test for protein and glucose, a check of the baby's heartbeat, and a measurement of fundal height (the size of the uterus as measured on the outside, along the belly, with an actual tape measure). Others will involve tests to check on the baby's development and your well-being. Here's a list of tests and approximately when they'll occur in your pregnancy:

At about 10 weeks: One or two genetic blood tests: the first trimester screening and noninvasive prenatal testing (NIPT), which can tell the gender (to be confirmed by ultrasound in a couple of weeks).

At about 12 weeks: A sonogram to confirm the due date, to look for twins, and to check on the placenta.

At about 16 weeks: A blood test for alpha-fetoprotein to screen for spina bifida, a defect of the spinal cord.

At about 20 weeks: An anatomy sonogram, which the doctor uses to check on important structures including the heart, spine, kidneys, brain, limbs, face, and more.

At about 26 weeks: A blood test for gestational diabetes and anemia.

At about 32 weeks: A sonogram to check the baby's weight and position.

At about 36 weeks: A vaginal swab for Group B strep infection (GBS) to indicate whether you'll need antibiotics in labor.

ABOUT INVASIVE TESTING

The question of whether to do invasive testing to confirm that your baby's genes are normal is complex and personal. There are a lot of factors, and the field of genetic testing—noninvasive (like blood tests) and invasive—is constantly advancing. There's a blood test between weeks 10 and 12 that identifies fetal DNA and provides high-quality screening for some of the more common chromosomal abnormalities like Down syndrome. Then there are optional invasive tests: CVS or amniocentesis. These tests involve inserting a needle into the uterus and gently obtaining cells from either the placenta or the fluid surrounding the baby. CVS (which happens around week 10) and amnio (between weeks 15 and 20) are highly accurate in identifying many types of genetic abnormalities—many more than blood tests can see—but they come with a risk of miscarriage (about a 1 in 500 chance). Age, family history, and other factors may come into play in the decision whether or not to do invasive testing. Your doctor or a genetic counselor can explain more in the context of your own pregnancy, which can be really helpful.

CAN I STAY ON MY MEDS?

With antidepressants and anti-anxiety meds, it's a case-by-case question that depends on the severity of the situation, the type of meds, and a few other factors. Let your caregiver know what meds you're taking as early as possible (ideally before you get pregnant). Celexa, Zoloft, Prozac, and Lexapro are among the antidepressants prescribed during pregnancy. If you're on something that's not safe during pregnancy, the doctor might work with your psychopharmacologist to switch you to a different drug. We monitor patients with depression closely because they're at increased risk for postpartum depression and anxiety. A postpartum doula—different from a labor doula, she comes in to help new parents in the early days—can make a difference; sleep is really important for combating depression and anxiety, and a postpartum doula (or friends and family) can help you get sleep. If you're under extreme stress, please tell your doctor or reach out to a therapist for support.

TELL YOUR DOCTOR

It's hard to know what might be relevant during pregnancy, so it's best to lay all your cards on the table. You'll be prompted on a range of topics when a staffer takes your medical history, but also be sure tell the doctor:

- if you or your partner is currently experiencing a stressful major life event.

- if you're on any medications (thyroid meds, for example, may need to be adjusted).

- if you're taking any supplements, herbs, or tinctures—regardless of how natural or innocuous they might seem.

- if your partner is taking any medication (Propecia, for male hair loss, for example, because you shouldn't touch the actual Propecia pill while pregnant).

- if you've ever been diagnosed with anxiety, depression, or an eating disorder.

- if you've traveled to Zika territory in the past three months or have plans to travel there during your pregnancy.

- anything that feels important to you about your own medical history or that of your parents or siblings.

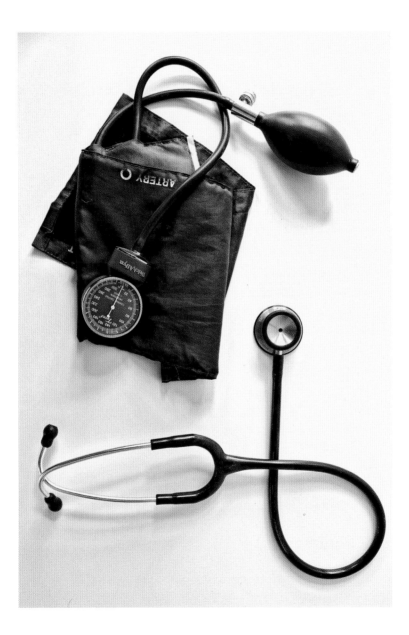

CHANGING PROVIDERS

If you feel like you're with the wrong practice, don't let it nag at you. You should be able to get your questions answered and be comfortable in the relationship. Talk to your doctor, give her a chance to address your concerns, and if the relationship still feels off, make a move. Sooner is better. You don't want to get locked in if it's not a fit. Some doctors won't take on new patients after 20 weeks. They want to be able to shepherd you all the way through your pregnancy—to keep an eye on you from the start. Once you determine you're in the right place, though, keep in mind that things are not always going to be perfect (just like in the rest of life). The most important thing to remember is that while your doctor wants you to have a good experience, her main concern is the well-being of you and your baby.

GET A FLU SHOT

When you're pregnant, your immune system is turned down a bit (which keeps your body from rejecting the baby as a foreign object), so if you get the flu, it can be more severe. In addition to the fact that you don't want to challenge your body to fight a strong illness while it's making a baby, the symptoms of flu—nausea, vomiting, fever, diarrhea—can cause you to become dehydrated, which can bring on premature labor. Confirm with your doctor first, and get a flu shot (not the nasal spray, though) anytime in pregnancy. The antibodies from your immunization will also protect your newborn. Also talk to your doctor about getting a T-Dap (tetanus, diptheria, pertussis) vaccine after 27 weeks to give the baby immunity to whooping cough.

YOU CAN ALWAYS CALL

Don't be shy about contacting your doctor with a concern. That's what she's there for. Please call in case of:

- vaginal bleeding
- leaking fluid
- severe abdominal or pelvic pain
- regular contractions
- decreased fetal movement
- inability to urinate
- inability to hold down food or fluids for twenty-four hours
- less frequent urination than normal
- darker than normal urine
- weight loss of 5 or more pounds in a week
- leg swelling or pain in one or both legs
- sudden severe puffiness of the hands or face
- severe headache
- light-headedness or faintness

- vomiting
- itching all over the body or on the hands and soles of the feet
- rash all over the body
- diarrhea lasting more than twenty-four hours
- burning when urinating
- fever or chills
- chest pain or shortness of breath
- abrupt onset of blurry vision or other sudden visual changes
- disturbing thoughts of hurting yourself or other people, or if you feel unsafe for any reason

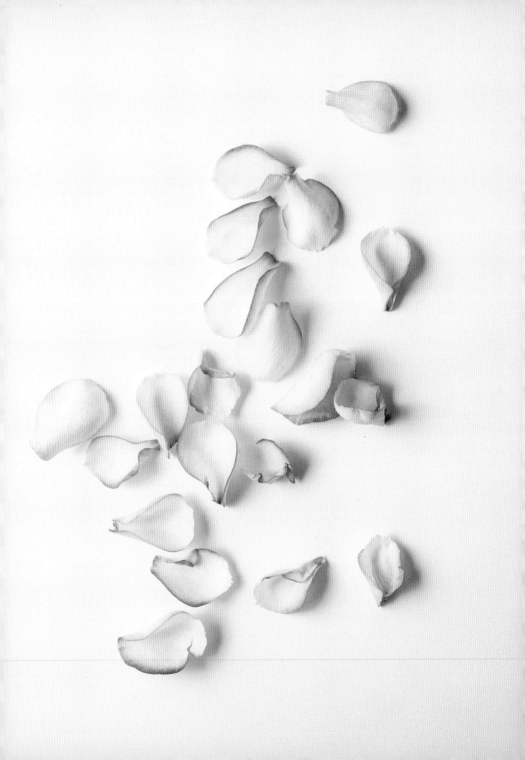

AN EMOTIONAL TOPIC

Some pregnancies don't make it. This, of course, can be crushing. Studies show that for some people, the grief of pregnancy loss can be just as bad for first-trimester miscarriages as for those at full term; other people might experience it as a normal process, as nature attempts to ensure a healthy baby. There's no "correct" way to feel or to process it. For the vast majority of people who miscarry, there's a problem with the meeting of the particular egg and sperm. It usually doesn't point to any problems with either parent. And it doesn't mean you won't have a normal pregnancy next time. If it happens, it's not your fault; resist the temptation to analyze everything you did leading up to that moment. An extra challenge if you find yourself in this situation is that people try to say the right thing, and sometimes it's the wrong thing, like "Everything happens for a reason" or "It's a blessing in disguise." Our culture doesn't have a great way to deal with pregnancy loss. We recommend talking with a therapist, especially one who has experience in this area, or seeing what support might be available through a nearby bereavement program. Feel your feelings—they're valid, whatever they might be.

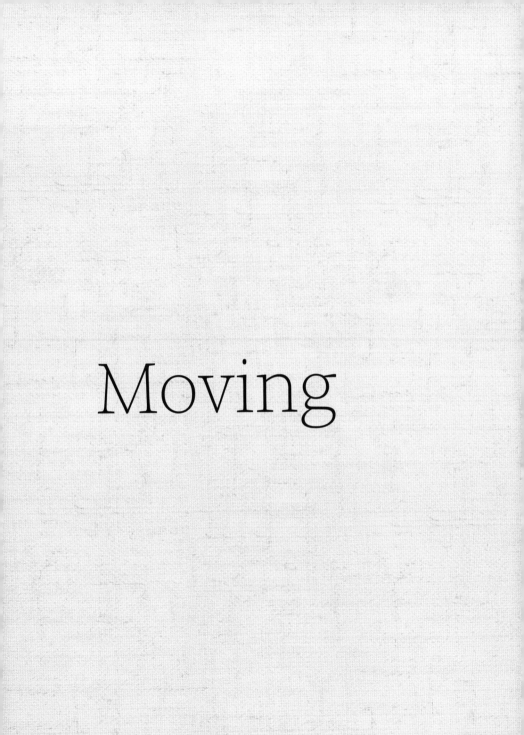

Moving

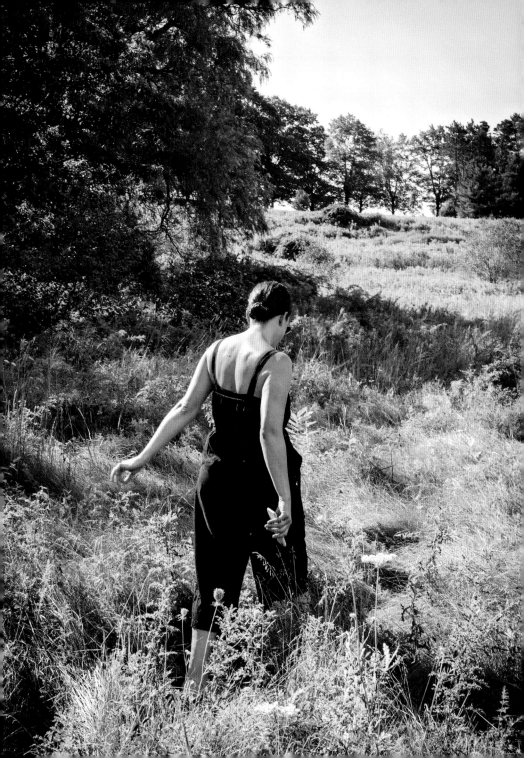

LISTEN TO YOUR BODY

During the first trimester, most reasonable exercise is fine as long as you're already used to it (don't take up running now for the first time ever). Aside from recommending a couple of adjustments—no inversions in yoga, no hot yoga—your doctor is likely to tell you to keep doing what you're doing. But your body might be saying something else. Something like, *Lie down*. Pay attention. You might need to dial it way back for a while, especially if you're experiencing a lot of nausea and/or exhaustion. If you don't feel up to your usual fitness commitments, take walks on a light incline, stretch when you wake up, or stream a gentle yoga class (try YogaGlo.com) and do only the poses you feel like doing. Your energy will most likely return soon.

NEW RULES OF FITNESS

Exercise is important in pregnancy. It helps your circulation, improves sleep, reduces stress, increases energy, and can minimize back pain, which lots of expectant mothers experience. Staying active can also lower your risk of gestational diabetes, Cesarean birth, and pre-eclampsia. After the first trimester, take a break from jarring activities or anything that comes with a risk of a fall: biking, running, skiing, racquet sports, horseback riding, jumping jacks (or anything else bouncy, like trampolines). This doesn't mean you can't work up a sweat or enjoy an endorphin high. Just take a lower-impact way there—spinning (as long as the room is not too hot), swimming (in a very clean pool), prenatal yoga, uphill walking (a 10-percent incline on the treadmill or something comparable outside). Aim for thirty minutes a day of moderate activity five (or more) times a week—walking counts. If you take a class that's longer than thirty minutes, that's fine, as long as there's an ebb and flow to the workout—we don't want you feeling faint (when you're pregnant, your blood sugar can drop more easily). As for intensity, you should be able to speak while exercising, and as pregnancy advances, you should reduce intensity. Even if you're very athletic, warm up and cool down. Drink lots of water before, during, and after workouts. Replace worn-out sneakers so you have lots of cushioning and support. Wear a well-fitting maternity bra and, when the time comes, maybe a maternity support belt. Because blood volume increases in pregnancy and your heart works harder to keep that blood circulating, you can become short of breath. This isn't the time to push your limits. The pregnancy hormone relaxin loosens joints, ligaments, and tendons, so it can be easier to injure yourself when you're pregnant, especially with workouts that focus on speed. Slower, more conscious types of movement—or programs designed especially for pregnant women—are a better choice. After 20 weeks, don't lie on your back while exercising. If your pregnancy is high risk, if you're expecting twins, or if you have cervical insufficiency or any other medical condition, talk to your doctor before exercising. And always stop exercising if you feel dizzy or light-headed, if you have signs of dehydration, or if something just doesn't feel right.

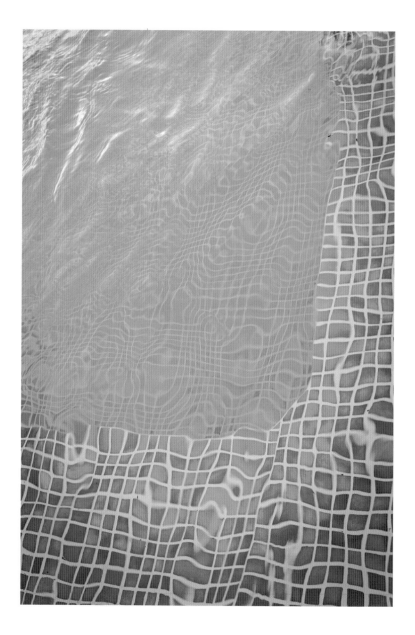

WORK OUT IN
CLEAN ENVIRONMENTS

You want to protect yourself from germs during pregnancy. Wipe off gym equipment before you use it. Bring your own yoga mat to class, as opposed to renting or borrowing a mat from the studio. Wear flip-flops in the locker room and shower. Swimming is good for your body, because it's gentle on joints, but you may be concerned about germs and chemicals. There are no good studies on chlorine absorption through pool swimming. Please swim only if you have access to a very clean, well-maintained pool. The water should not smell heavily of chlorine (scoop up a handful and give it a sniff). Use common sense, plus a little extra caution. Wash hands well before you eat anything after a workout. If a gym or a studio feels unclean or underventilated, don't go there. We don't want to make you crazy, just conscious.

DOES EXERCISE HELP
WITH LABOR?

Labor can be a bit of a marathon, so in a way, endurance exercise—swimming laps or spinning, for example— might make you feel more prepared. But this is much more of a mental preparation than a physical one. Your uterus is a muscle but not one you can strengthen or train. It functions involuntarily. Working out in pregnancy is not about preparing that muscle for action. It's about keeping your body healthy and your blood moving. But the same fortitude that in the past has gotten you through, say, a grueling set of push-ups can come into play when you're powering through painful contractions. Any practice you've had in pushing your body well past its comfort zone will serve you in the delivery room, where it's largely about stamina. Women who exercise also have, on average, slightly shorter labors (by about fifty minutes).

DO YOUR KEGELS
(AND REVERSE KEGELS)

The pelvic floor is buoyant—a hammock of muscles capable of moving up and down. You've heard about Kegel exercises to strengthen this area. We recommend combining them with *reverse* Kegels to stretch and relax the muscles—that's what your body needs to do during labor to move the baby out. For Kegels, lift and tighten the pelvic floor muscles for a count of five, then relax and repeat. It's the same group of muscles that stops the stream of urine. The feeling is up and in. A reverse Kegel is the opposite—down and out. It's subtle, so don't worry if you can't quite feel it. To get in touch with the sensation, take a big inhale—feel how the muscles of the pelvic floor naturally drop? Try to maintain that feeling for a count of five. You can combine Kegels and reverse Kegels so that you pull up and hold for five seconds, then drop down for five seconds and hold. Work your way up to ten-second holds. Do three sets a day, ten reps each set, starting in the second trimester. These exercises can not only help prevent urinary leakage in pregnancy and aid you in pushing out the baby but can also make a difference later, when it comes to sex, orgasm, and minimizing postpartum leaking.

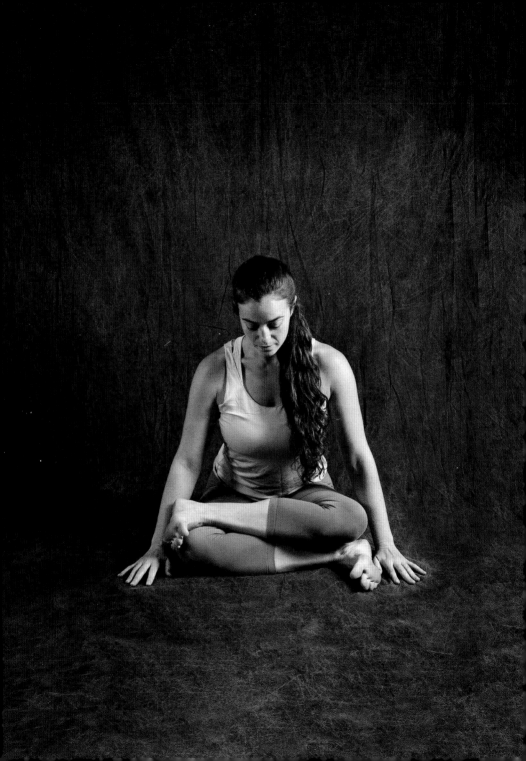

WHAT'S DIFFERENT ABOUT
PRENATAL YOGA?

Prenatal yoga classes tend to skip inversions, closed twists, backbends, positions that have you lying on your back—and other stuff we'd rather you not do when pregnant. It's nice to be in a class that's designed to look after your well-being and that errs on the side of caution. Flowing through asanas is better than holding poses for a long time; stasis is not great, as we mentioned (see page 46). No Bikram or other forms of hot yoga, please. Use props—blocks, blankets, bolsters—to make yourself comfortable. If you're already a yogi, we don't have to sell you on yoga's benefits. It can be so helpful in pregnancy, slowing your heart rate, lowering blood pressure, aiding in circulation, lifting your mood, decreasing anxiety, and serving as a balm for achy joints and muscles. You might miss the bliss of headstands, but you can still enjoy a whole-body practice and all the benefits of linking breath to movement. On the following pages are some of the poses recommended during pregnancy.

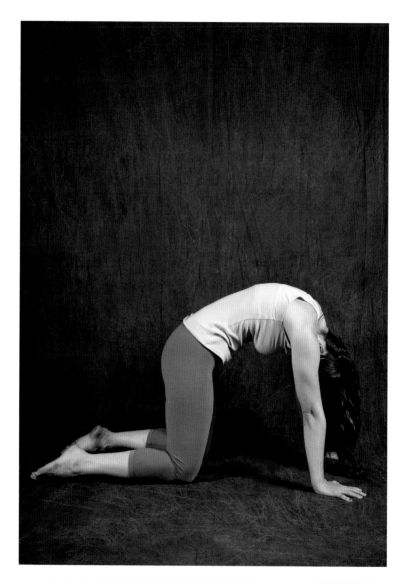

Cat-Cow pose—moving between the rounded shape above and a gentle arch opens the upper back and chest, engages the triceps, and invites your neck and shoulder muscles to let go. Turn your fingers the other way to release your wrists (great if you're at a keyboard all day).

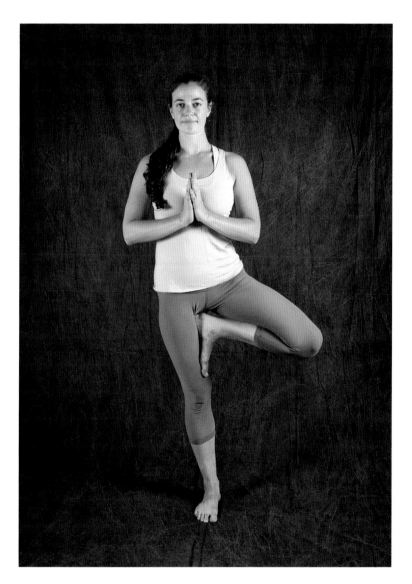

Tree pose is customizable. The lifted foot can be wherever it's comfortable—against the thigh as shown, against the calf, or resting on the ankle (but don't press it against the knee, please).

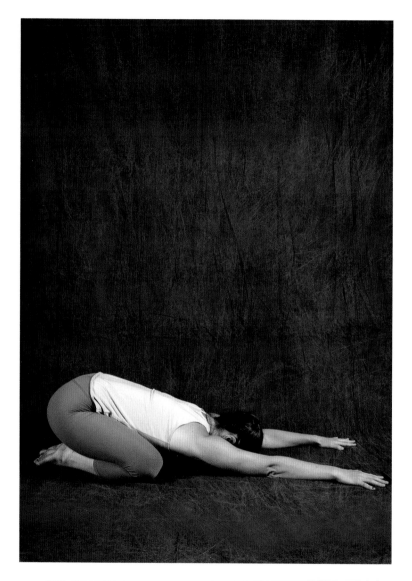

Wide-knee Child's pose leaves room for a belly. Creep fingers forward to stretch shoulders or relax elbows down for more of a resting pose.

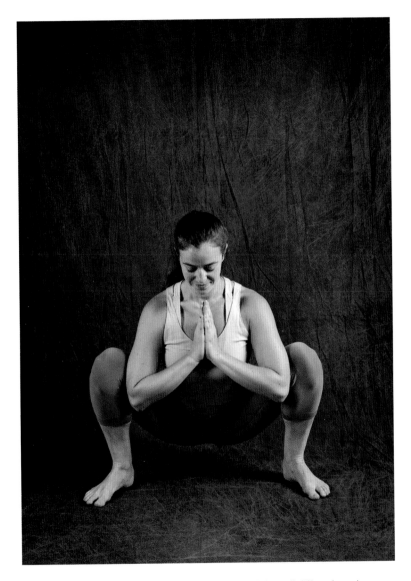

Squat pose broadens the lower back and can bring relief if you're achy there. Tuck a yoga block under your seat for support if you like.

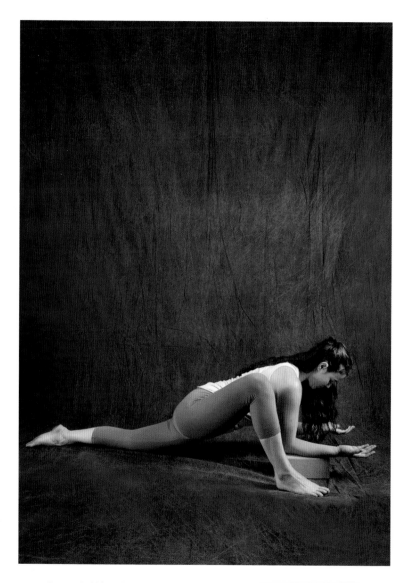

Supported Lizard pose releases the hips, and can feel great on the inner thigh if you let that front knee open a bit.

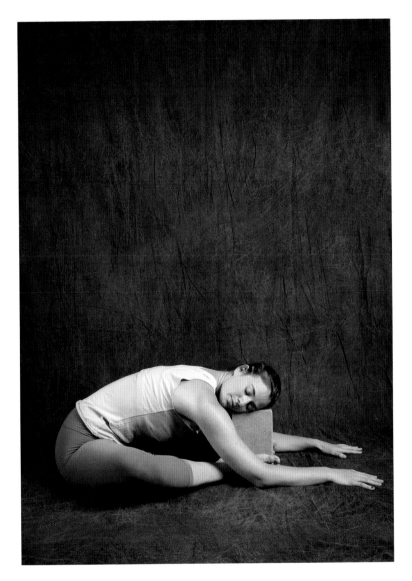

Supported Star pose gives you another way to rest. If your knees need some support, just stick a rolled-up towel beneath each. A block between your feet is grounding and feels great.

Comfort & Relaxation

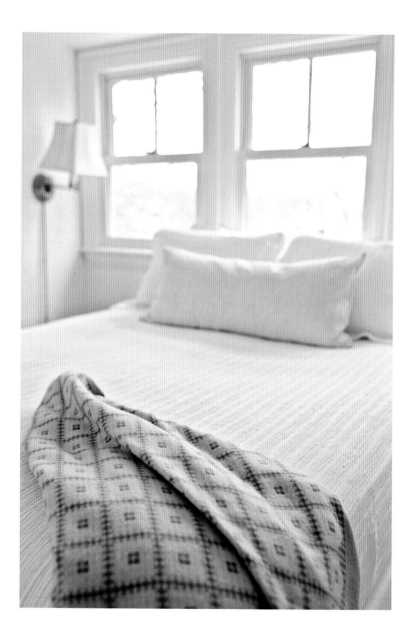

TAKE SLEEP LIKE A VITAMIN

One of the easiest ways to take care of yourself while pregnant is to make sleep a priority. Your body, in the first trimester, puts in a clear request for this; the exhaustion can be epic. Don't fight it. Just lie down when you can. It's a luxury afforded first-time moms. If there's a day or a week or even a month you can't imagine going to the gym, head home and nap instead. At night, for the best possible sleep, keep the bedroom cool and totally dark—cover blinking lights with black tape. Don't bring screens to bed. Leave your phone to charge in another room so you're not tempted (get an alarm clock if you normally use your phone to wake up). Your bedroom will feel so much more restful without it. As pregnancy advances, swap sides of the bed if that gives you easier access to the bathroom, and toss out the snorer next to you on occasion if the noise interferes with your REM sleep. Sleep helps keep your stress level down and makes it much easier to maintain the nutritious diet you need—when you're tired, your body cries out for carbs and sugar.

ROSE, LAVENDER, CHAMOMILE

Essential oils made from herbs and flowers can be powerful, so don't mess around with random potions when you're pregnant. After the first trimester, a few safe oils you can enjoy—and add to a bath—are rose, lavender, chamomile, ylang-ylang, and mandarin. Erbaviva organic massage oil is nice for achy muscles. As we've mentioned, some people find the fragrance of peppermint or lemongrass to be a nice natural antidote to nausea—you can buy a roll-on oil meant for pregnancy and dab it on your wrist. With any oils, opt for those that are certified organic—there's no way to know what synthetic versions contain—and use them in a diluted form (just a couple of drops in a bath); they can be very potent and may irritate already sensitive pregnant skin.

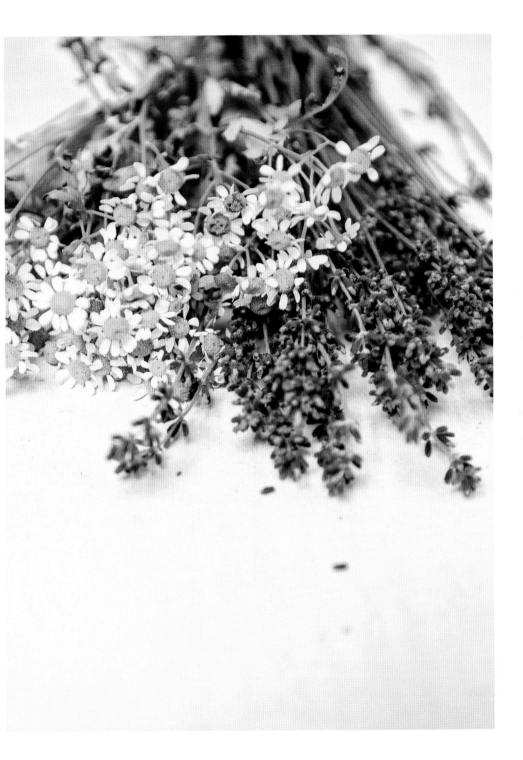

IF YOUR BACK IS ACHY OR YOUR PELVIS HURTS

Musculoskeletal problems like back pain and pelvic pressure are common due to extra weight and changes in posture, especially as you move into the later part of the second trimester. A maternity belt can really help. It's a cozy, wide band that hugs you gently around the hips, adding support below the belly. It stabilizes joints—which are loosened by the hormone relaxin— and improves overall comfort. Use the maternity belt during exercise and while you're at work. Some lifestyle adjustments can also help. If you tend to lug around a big shoulder bag, swap it for a smallish backpack and shorten the straps to keep the weight against your body. Consciously engage your thighs and abs when walking up stairs, and get up from your desk to stretch the lower back with a yoga squat now and then (see page 121). You can also find relief in treatments like prenatal massage (safe in all three trimesters), prenatal acupuncture, prenatal acupressure, and prenatal chiropractic care.

NO WINE, NO WEED

Absolutely do not smoke cigarettes or vape (or inhale secondhand smoke) while you're pregnant. When it comes to pot . . . well, just in case there's confusion or a gray area with forms that don't involve inhaling (such as edibles or CBD oil), we want to be clear: Weed crosses the placenta, and its effect on babies is not yet known, so don't use it in any form when you're pregnant. As for wine and other alcohol, skip it; we just don't know if there's an absolute amount that's safe, so it's best not to drink at all. Don't freak yourself out if you drank or smoked before you knew you were pregnant. But once you're on the path to growing a baby, stay clean. You'll spend the vast majority of your life *not* pregnant and able to do whatever you want. During this special time, err on the side of safety.

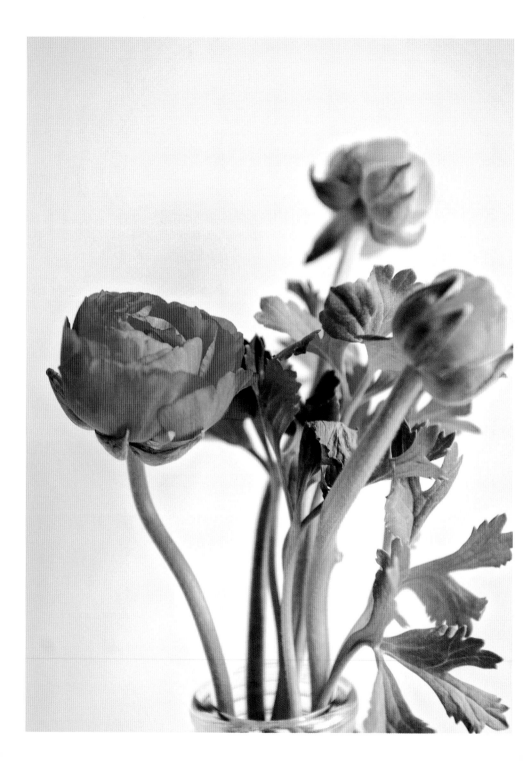

KEEP IT POSITIVE

You're going to lose personal space when you're pregnant. Getting on an elevator with a big belly is like walking down the street with an adorable puppy. People will smile and try to catch your eye. Some might try to touch you. Obviously, this is crossing a line, and nobody should touch your body without asking (you can shut it down with a simple "I'd rather you didn't"). But it might happen. People's reactions to pregnancy are primal, and it can be helpful to remind yourself of that. You're part of something bigger now, a universal experience that makes strangers feel connected. If you can enjoy and embrace this, you'll probably feel more relaxed. Same holds true when it comes to unasked-for advice. From predictions about what gender your baby is to opinions on what you happen to be eating in that moment, input abounds. People want to share their stories and reexperience that time in their own lives. This can occasionally go off the rails, and in that case, take care of yourself. If you cross paths with a gloom-and-doomer who free-associates toward some tale of tragedy, halt the conversation. Just say, "I'm trying to be really positive—that's what my doctor wants me to do."

TRY TO SLEEP ON YOUR SIDE

While it's true that you want to avoid long periods on your back from 22 weeks on, it's really more of an issue when you're awake. At night, your body naturally rolls over or wakes you up if you've been on your back too long. If you're generally healthy and have an uncomplicated pregnancy, don't worry about moving around in the night (and don't sacrifice a good night's sleep to keep rebuilding the pillow fort that keeps you on your side). Side positions maximize blood flow to the placenta, helping to keep circulation nice and easy. Lying on your right side is just as good as lying on your left side, it turns out—and a great night's sleep is best of all. When you're awake and in charge—reading in bed, exercising, or stretched out on the sofa watching TV—make a conscious effort to switch from side to side and minimize flat-back lounging.

STAY THERMONEUTRAL

That's an interesting way of saying no saunas, steam rooms, hot tubs, hot yoga, or superhot baths (a bath so hot it makes you sweat). High heat can adversely affect the embryo's neural tube development (spinal cord and brain). You generally want to stay in thermoneutral environments while you're pregnant. Don't worry about exercise—it doesn't increase the temperature of your body in the same way. But no diving into icy waters for a New Year's Day ritual, throwing yourself into the snow after a sweat-lodge awakening (double no), or spending the night in an ice hotel. Not too hot, not too cold.

MEDITATE (OR JUST BREATHE)

If meditation sounds like homework, just take a minute now and then to enjoy five slow, full, conscious breaths. On your commute, in an elevator, on line at the supermarket, it's a simple way to release and a great habit to cultivate. Meditation itself doesn't have to be formal or lengthy. Here's a quickie to squeeze in anytime: Rest your hands in your lap and close your eyes softly. Focus on your sense of hearing and let your breath naturally settle and expand. Let the ambient sounds come to you—don't work too hard. Just passively take in what's there. Voices, the hum of the heat or air conditioner, traffic, music, birds (after 19 weeks, your baby can hear these outside sounds too). Allow your attention to rest where it naturally goes or let it flit from sound to sound—there's no wrong way to do this. Deepen your breath and check to see that your jaw is released. How are your shoulders? Let them melt. Stay as long as you like. When you're ready to come back, flutter your eyes a little bit to ease reentry.

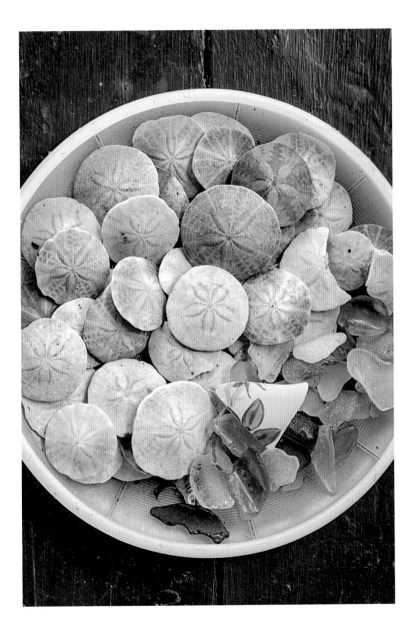

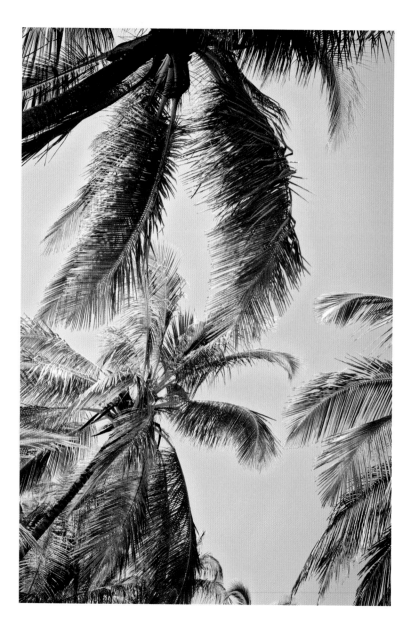

NEW RULES OF VACATION

Skip vacation activities that could cause a fall, like riding horses or mopeds, surfing, skiing, or playing in rough waters. Don't visit altitudes above 6,000 feet (if you're struggling to breathe, it puts both you and the baby at risk), and no scuba. Pass on cruises—too many germs, such as norovirus. In general, keep yourself out of harm's way. When you're not sure about a certain activity or food, opt out. If there are insects around (this applies at home too), use a product containing 10 to 35 percent DEET. During pregnancy, the risks associated with certain types of insect bites are far worse than those associated with chemical bug repellent. But do your best to cover up with long sleeves, long pants, and a hat. Don't go anyplace where there are food- or waterborne infections. Obviously, don't go where there's Zika. If your partner travels to Zika territory while you're pregnant, do not have unprotected sex for the entire pregnancy. Got that? Zika can live in the semen. You can use condoms and have sex, but no unprotected sex till the baby is born. (If you're reading this book in advance of pregnancy and you or your partner has recently been to Zika territory, wait three months to become pregnant.)

FLYING PREGNANT

Some doctors ask patients not to fly in the first trimester simply because that's when the chance of miscarriage is highest (while flying won't cause a miscarriage, you don't want that to happen on a plane or on a trip). Once you're cleared for air travel, be vigilant about taking care of yourself in the air. Pregnancy raises your risk of blood clots (see page 57). Air travel also independently raises the risk of blood clots. So the combination of air travel and pregnancy is something to take seriously. There's also a higher risk of dehydration in air travel in general, and this is much more significant in pregnancy (it puts you at risk for preterm labor and is another risk factor for clotting). Please take the following precautions:

- Buy two huge bottles of water for the flight (don't depend on the drinks carts and those tiny cups).

- Change your leg position as much as space allows (uncross and cross legs, contract and release muscles).

- Consider wearing compression stockings on the plane; the support prevents blood from pooling in your legs.

- Get up and walk around the plane as often as you can (get the blood moving).

- Stretch while waiting for the restroom (where you will be often, because of all the water you're drinking).

We suggest caution with air travel within two months of your due date (at that point, in the event that your baby is born early, he would likely be okay with the help of the services at a hospital). Even though you're unlikely to go into labor this early, if it should happen, you don't want to be giving birth in the air—or even in a place that's not home. A newborn's immune system is vulnerable, and the germy environment of an airplane poses some risk, so your pediatrician may not want you to fly home right away. In those last couple of months, it's a good idea to stay local.

Homestretch

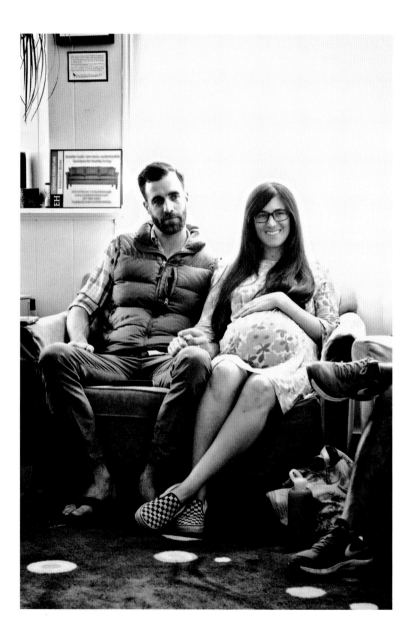

FIND A BIRTHING CLASS

Prenatal classes can be sweet and meaningful—very special date nights for you and your partner. Ask your caregiver or doula for suggestions. This ensures a good philosophical fit, but don't stress about it—Lamaze, Bradley, Alexander, and other methods all prepare you well. Aim to start your class at about 30 weeks. If you can find a small class in an intimate environment, all the better. Make the time to get to class in a relaxed way, and be attentive students. You'll be surprised how often the nuggets you've gleaned will pop up to help you later on. If your schedules are insane and it's really difficult to make this happen, do online classes together at your convenience. It's better to enjoy and focus on these lessons as a happy interlude than to make yourselves stressed trying to get to the live-action version. Lamaze .org and other sites offer online courses.

WATCH NURSING VIDEOS

As you'll discover, in some ways nursing is the most natural thing in the world, but the technical aspects are imitative skills. It's really teachable. So this is one of those rare times we encourage you to go online. Search "how to breastfeed" on YouTube. Watching a baby latch on to a breast over and over gets your eye used to what you're aiming for—which is the baby opening wide and taking in the whole areola, not just the nipple (more on this on page 203). It's pretty amazing—and in watching videos, you might see how instinctive it is for babies to do this "right." If you're having any anxiety about nursing, getting a good look at the technique can help build your confidence. Some patients ask if there's anything special they should do predelivery to prep breasts for nursing. There's nothing you need to do. You're ready for it.

STRETCH THAT PERINEUM

Gentle self-administered perineal massage makes a huge difference in vaginal delivery and recovery. It sets you up for a better birth experience, with less vaginal tearing and less chance of an episiotomy. Give it a few minutes a day, starting at 34 weeks. The area you want to focus on is the perineum, which includes the skin and the strong horizontal muscle along the bottom of the vagina. Find the best position for you—this might be sitting up in bed propped on pillows, with your knees bent, or lying on your side. Make sure your hands are clean and your nails are short. Use lubricant (non-petroleum based, such as Weleda Perineum Massage Oil, or just olive oil). Insert your thumbs or two fingers about an inch into the vagina and apply pressure at the "six o'clock" spot. Then move your fingers toward nine o'clock and three o'clock while gently massaging tissue. Repeat this motion, stopping now and then to hold the stretched positions at nine and three. Continue for about five minutes. Don't press so hard that you're in pain (you might feel a little burning the first week or two). When possible, do your perineal massage after a warm bath, when tissue is more supple.

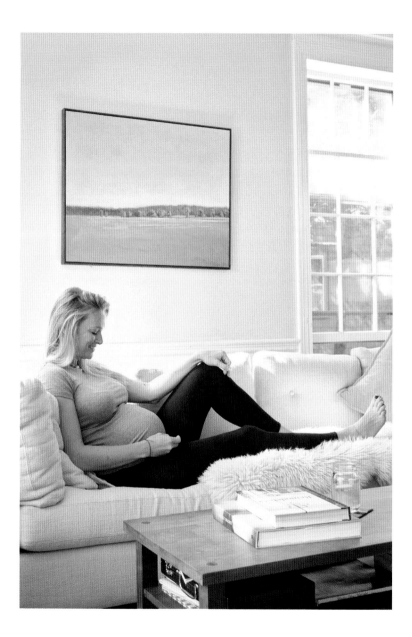

CHECKING IN ON THE BABY'S MOVEMENT

Starting at about 28 weeks, sit down daily at a time you know the baby tends to be active, and take note of the baby's movements. If you're not feeling anything right away, have a cold drink or a few bites of something sweet—that tends to get the baby going. You want to feel ten movements within two hours (you might easily feel ten movements in ten minutes—in that case, you're all done counting). Later in pregnancy, when the baby gains most of her weight, there's less space inside for moving around, so activity can feel a bit subtler. What's important is that you get to know your baby's patterns so you're aware if there's a decrease in activity. If you don't feel ten movements in two hours—or if you're ever worried about decreased fetal movement for any reason—don't wait; call your doctor.

BIG SISTERS AND BROTHERS

If you have one of these at home waiting for her or his new baby, there are a couple of small things you can do to help make the meeting of the siblings smooth and positive. In the hospital, tape a little photo of your older child inside the baby's bassinet, so when your big kid comes, she sees herself with her baby right away, and knows the baby has been "looking at" her. You also might want to have the baby in the bassinet when your bigger child arrives, so your arms are free to hug your older child. She and your partner can wheel the baby to you. It can help give your older child a sweet sense of ownership. When you come home from the hospital, same note. Walk through the door with your arms free for a hug; your partner can enter behind you, carrying the baby.

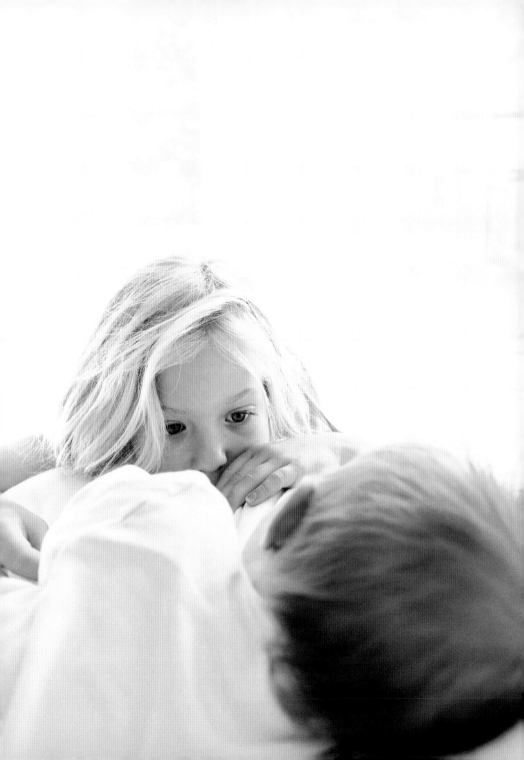

WRITING YOUR BIRTH PLAN

You don't have to be formal and businesslike in a birth plan. Think of it as a letter to your medical team. Feel free to be yourself. Some of our patients begin with an expression of gratitude ("We're thankful to be delivering at General Hospital . . . ") and convey an understanding that safety comes first. Here are some of the requests we often see, plus some we recommend. Most everything here is described elsewhere in the book. Pick and choose and add your own. You can lead into your list with something like "I am hoping to have":

- an unmedicated birth/an epidural available to me immediately/the chance to go as far as possible without an epidural and then have one available.

- a medlock for the IV so I can move around easily.

- my birthing ball with me at the hospital.

- access to nitrous oxide (sometimes called gas and air), if the hospital uses it.

- skin-to-skin contact immediately after delivery for as much of the first hour as possible, with newborn procedures performed while the baby is on me, and others delayed till after the first hour.

- help nursing as soon as possible.

- delayed cord clamping.

- in the event of a C-section, as much help as possible to have skin-to-skin contact in the operating room and possibly breastfeed. I don't want anything to interfere with the safe performance of surgery, but I would like . . .

  the IV placed so I can bend an arm to hold the baby.

  the EKG leads on my back or side instead of on my chest.

  the pulse monitor clipped to my ear instead of my finger.

  my arms free of the gown.

At about 32 weeks, bring the birth plan to your doctor's appointment. Ask the doctor to give it a look, and take notes while she comments. Hospital policy may knock out a few of your asks. Edit accordingly, and then you have a short, sweet, well-thought-out document to bring to the hospital on the big day.

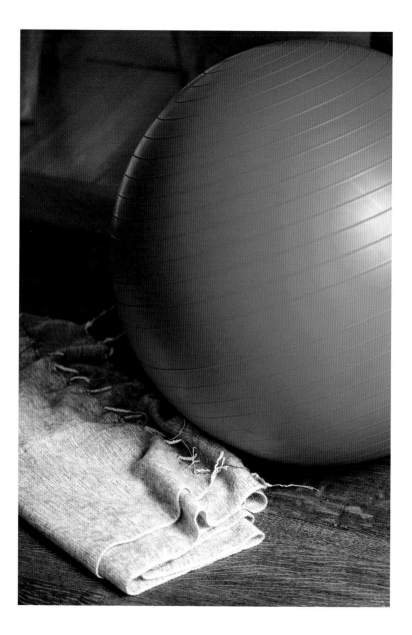

GET A BIRTHING BALL

In labor, switching positions is what keeps you going. A big exercise ball—aka a birthing ball—can help. Have one at home for early labor, and ask your doctor if you can bring it to the hospital (also include this in your birth plan). The ball provides soft, flexible support. You can sit on it with your feet flat and your torso resting on your partner, relax on the floor in a wide kneel and rest your upper body on the ball, recline on it momentarily to release tightness in the front of your body—it's an all-purpose assist. Get the right size so you're safe and secure while seated (there are two sizes: the 65-centimeter ball is recommended for those shorter than 5 foot 8, and the 75-centimeter for those taller). If you're bringing your ball to the hospital, confirm in advance that it fits in your car or buy a second one that you can leave in the box uninflated, so it's easy to pack and transport. Check to make sure that all parts are present and in working order: ball, pump, pin, stopper.

WHAT YOU NEED
FOR A NEWBORN

Your due date can feel like a hard deadline by which you must do a million things in order to be READY FOR THE BABY. The truth is, you need very little for a newborn, and you have plenty of time to get the rest. At first, all you need is your body, a bassinet, diapers, some cotton onesies, muslin squares or cloth diapers as burp cloths, Desitin ointment, a little soft hairbrush, a tiny nail clipper, soft small blankets, a car seat, a stroller, a baby bathtub, and a front carrier. What you don't need till later? A crib, an Exersaucer, a bouncy chair, a bedroom for the baby—truly, almost everything. Try not to get stressed out or fight with your partner over this. You might be nervous and tense about the big life change coming, and that can get channeled into concern over tangible items (it's so much easier to talk about the unassembled dresser than to dig into the deeper stuff). Let it go. Stay light and on the same team.

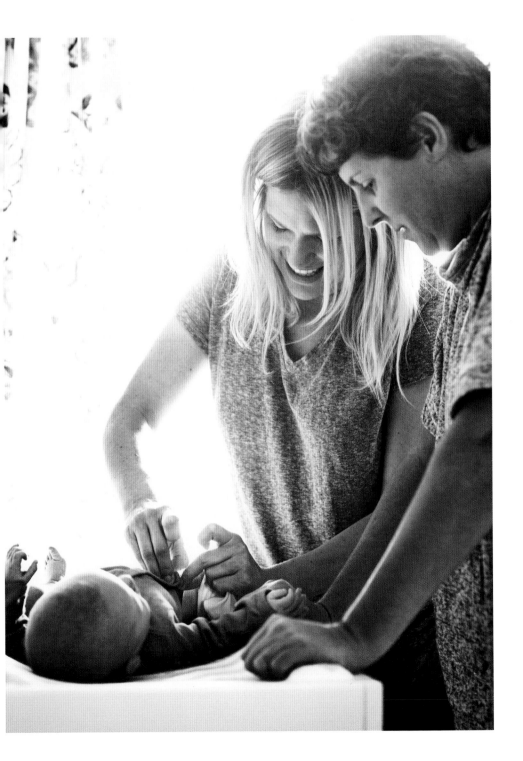

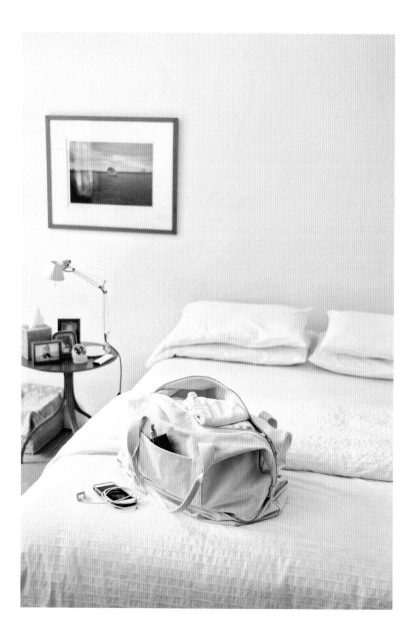

PACKING FOR THE HOSPITAL

At its simplest, bring yourself, your partner, your doula, your phone, your wallet (with ID and insurance cards), a labor outfit if you want to wear your own clothes (ask your doctor in advance if this is an option), your birthing ball, and your birth plan. Almost everything else can be provided or fetched later, after the birth. But here's a more complete list of some helpful items:

- button-front nightgown for nursing
- robe
- comfy clothes to go home in
- nursing bras
- breast pads
- toiletries/makeup/hairbrush
- glasses and contact lenses; lens case; saline solution
- Colgate Wisps—disposable mini toothbrushes that are preloaded with toothpaste (because you can't always get up to brush your teeth)
- facial cleansing wipes
- any meds you take, with the dosage

- slippers (that fit well and won't trip you)
- flip-flops (for the shower)
- lip balm
- hair bands
- magazines
- phone charger
- playlists/headphones/Bluetooth speaker
- snacks
- your favorite pillow
- eye mask (it can be bright in the hospital at night)
- baby clothes for the trip home
- elastic support garment (more on this on page 237)
- an infant car seat (if you have a car, install the car seat in back from the get-go—you can't take your baby home from the hospital without it; if you're traveling by cab, have a family member bring the car seat the day after you deliver)
- photos of your older child

MAP YOUR ROUTE

A few weeks before your due date, drive to the hospital (or take a cab if that's going to be your travel mode). In a relaxed way, take a peek at where you'll be going—drive to the drop-off area, navigate the parking lot. If it's permitted, take the elevator up to the labor and delivery floor (take an official tour, if one is offered). It's comforting to know what the place looks like, where to turn left or right, how many hallways you'll walk through till you get where you need to be. For those who live especially far from the hospital, there can be a lot of anxiety around getting there, especially with the possibility of traffic or bad weather. If you live very far, consider setting up an option for laboring nearby—maybe at the home of a friend or relative. Coming closer will make it easier for you to relax. The goal is to spend early labor at home or somewhere else comfortable—and not to go to the hospital too soon, as long as that's okay with your doctor. When people are anxious about the trip, they sometimes end up at the hospital too soon—and this can affect the way labor plays out.

GET YOUR PET READY

If you already have a baby of the canine or feline variety, there are a few things you can do in advance to help make the coming changes a little easier—and possibly to curtail stressful postpartum pet behaviors. If, for example, a certain room (or your bed) will be off-limits once the baby arrives, implement the rule in late pregnancy to give your pet time to get used to it (and get over it). You also want to acclimate your pet to the sensory experience of a newborn. Wash some of the baby's new clothes, and let your pet smell them. Play a recording of newborn noises every now and then (go to Calmsound.com, and look under Calm Pet: Desensitizing Sounds for Animals). Try not to smother your pet with love in anticipation of the new situation; give her a normal amount of attention. And before you come home from the hospital with the baby, have your partner bring home a blanket with the baby's scent for your pet to sniff.

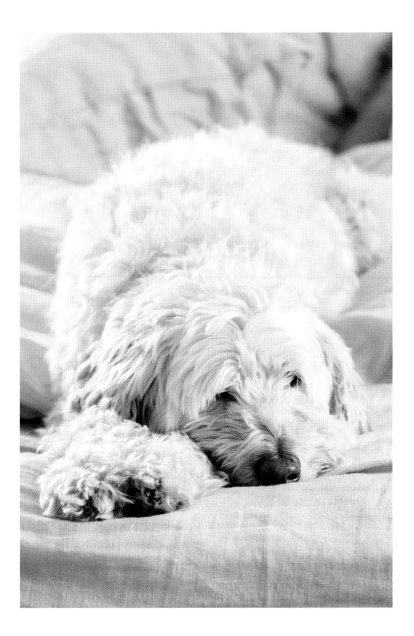

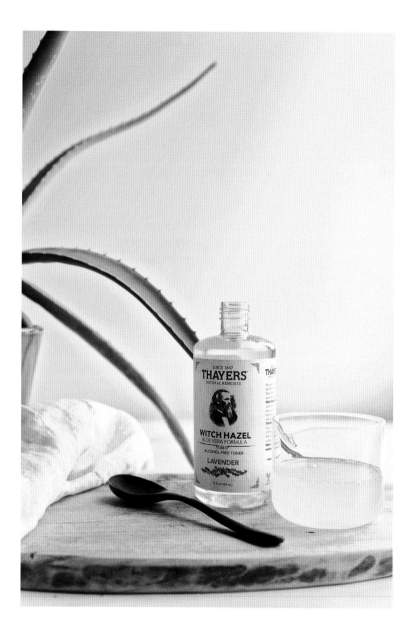

POSTPARTUM COOLING PADS

When you come home after a vaginal birth and discover these soothers in the freezer (after having forgotten you ever made them), you'll be ever-grateful to the nesting instinct responsible for such productivity. All you need to make postpartum cooling pads are a dozen or so unscented, chlorine-free maxi pads with wings—biggest size you can find (Seventh Generation Free & Clear Overnight, for example)—a bottle of witch hazel, organic aloe gel (Earth's Daughter Organic or Seven Minerals), and plastic freezer bags. Pour some witch hazel on the pads, top with a generous schmear of aloe gel, and zip each pad into its own plastic bag. Store in the freezer, and you're all set. Start making use of these postpartum pads as soon as you're back from the hospital. Your perineum will thank you.

THE ENDLESS END
OF PREGNANCY

Time can go so slowly those last weeks. Here's a reminder of some things you can do as you listen to the clock tick, tick, tick, and you wait, wait, wait for labor:

- Choose your pediatrician.
- Make a playlist for the hospital.
- Write thank-you emails for gifts you've received, even if you end up following up with paper cards.
- Cook and freeze some favorite foods.
- Meditate.
- Take walks with friends.
- Find out what your insurance company might cover postpartum—like a lactation consultant.
- Get a prenatal massage.
- Think about which contraceptive method you want to use postpartum (breastfeeding is not reliable as contraception).
- Think about whether you want to circumcise your baby if it's a boy.

- Learn infant CPR.

- Talk to friends with babies about how to find and interview potential child-care providers (this can be a postpartum stressor, and a little intel can help).

Some things you *shouldn't* do right before labor:

- Get spa treatments that expose you to chemicals or immerse you in water.

- Shave your bikini area. This can make you more susceptible to infection.

- Begin DIY home projects you've been meaning to tackle that are stressful or complicated and involve ladders or chemicals—the nesting instinct can be strong, but this is a better time to sort socks.

- Take long car rides.

- Stress yourself out trying to get your entire life in order before the baby comes. Time will not stop. We promise.

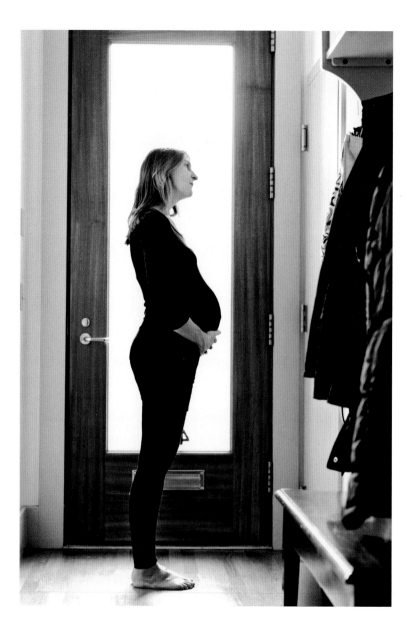

HAS THE BABY DROPPED?

People will ask you this question. You might wonder what exactly it refers to. It's a shift in the position of the baby that happens late in the third trimester. All of a sudden, you find you can breathe more easily—there's more space between the bottom of your rib cage and the uterus. It's not something everyone can see; it's something you *feel* first. The baby dropping is a sign that you're moving toward labor, but there's no time frame connected to it—as in, we still have no idea exactly when labor will start. It usually begins a couple of weeks after the baby drops. The doctor will check your uterus through your abdomen (just by touching) to determine the position of the baby. Some women choose to have a session with a prenatal chiropractor around week 34 to help them become more comfortable in those last weeks—our patients report that this helps a lot. The chiropractor helps align and balance the pelvis so the baby is in an ideal position, with the most room, which can really ease labor and delivery.

Laboring

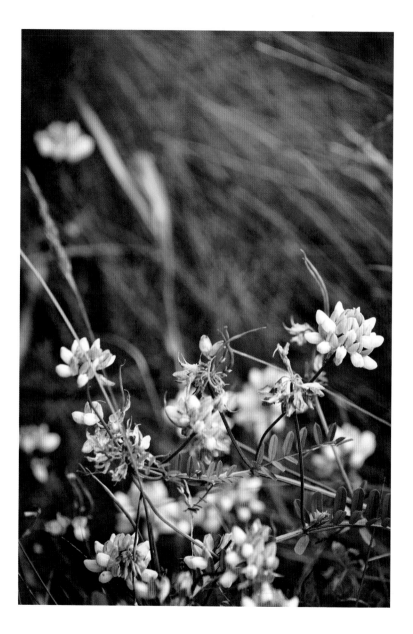

THE BIRTH PROCESS CAN START A FEW WAYS

Spontaneous labor is when your body begins the labor process on its own. Patients ask us all the time about natural ways to start labor (spicy food? walking? acupuncture?). Although there's no evidence that these methods work, you're welcome to try them. They won't harm you. Many patients tell us that sex hastens labor. Another option is an old technique called a membrane sweep, often done by midwives. The practitioner uses a finger to touch the lining of the cervix. She's not breaking the water, just sweeping her finger along the amniotic sac to separate it from the cervix. It's something your caregiver might do in an office visit near your due date.

Induction is a medical treatment that starts contractions for the safety of the mother and/or baby. At certain times it's necessary. It's a procedure that happens in the hospital, so you won't be laboring at home; you'll have a fetal monitor, which can make it harder to move around. But it doesn't have to be a big deal. It often involves medication to "ripen" the cervix (soften it and help it dilate) followed by an IV of Pitocin to jump-start contractions. If your doctor says she wants to induce labor, know why and how. Reasons for induction could include high blood pressure, gestational diabetes, concern about the baby's size, or concern about passing the due date. What induction is not for: getting around the holidays, timing the baby for when your mother can fly into town, or ensuring that you can be delivered by a certain doctor in your practice. If you're being induced, the beginning of your labor is going to be different—you'll be in the hospital, not at home—but by the time you get into active labor, it's all the same.

If your water breaks, even if you're not yet having contractions, things become time-sensitive. There are concerns, including infection, that come with a long time between water breaking and birth. You'll notify your doctor if and when your water breaks—let her know if your fluid is green or bloody. Then she can keep an eye on that clock for you, synthesize the specifics of your situation, and determine when you need to go to the hospital. First-time mothers sometimes worry that they won't know if their water has broken. If you're not sure—sometimes it's dramatic and other times more like a leak—call the doctor to be safe. Amniotic fluid smells sweet, not at all like urine.

A scheduled Cesarean birth might happen because of safety concerns or because you had a C-section before. Some women elect to have Cesarean births for personal reasons. Keep in mind that a C-section is surgery, and surgery comes with some risks. If you're considering a C-section because you think it will lead to a better sex life later, we want to share that data shows that after six months, sexual function is basically the same whether you've delivered vaginally or by C-section.

Talk to your doctor about what she'd like you to do when labor begins—get clear on her approach and any relevant guidelines from your hospital, so you're all on the same page and can relax about the logistics. The next few pages talk about strategies for early labor.

EARLY LABOR AT HOME

One of the things that can lead to a path of interventions in normal labor is showing up at the hospital too early. Many hospitals just aren't designed for early labor. During this phase, which can be long, you'll want to be moving around and soaking and walking and sipping and changing positions—so home is ideal. With a first baby, a lot of people head to the hospital too soon. What can happen then is the medicalizing of a very natural process. Protocol usually demands that you be attached to a fetal monitor and an IV as soon as you're at the hospital. At home, you can go for a walk, have a bite if you're hungry (keep it light and nutritious—nausea is common in labor), switch from chair to birthing ball to squat to yoga mat to sofa. You can sit on a sturdy folding chair in the shower and let the warm water run down your back. There are so many options for comfort and distraction, and this is what you need through early labor. Later, when your labor is stronger, you won't want to move around much—at that point, a small space feels right, and the hospital is a perfect place to be.

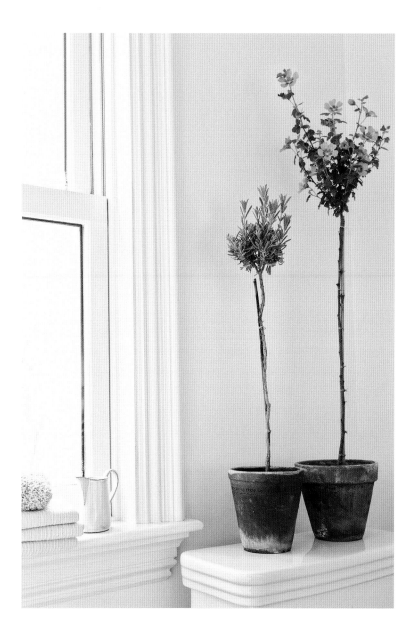

TIMINGWISE, THINK 5-1-1

If you're laboring at home, your caregiver will likely
want you to go to the hospital when labor is "real."
There's no precise formula for determining when labor
is real, but one rubric we use is "5-1-1": contractions that
are five minutes apart, each lasting for one minute, with
this pattern continuing for at least one hour. Of course,
the uterus doesn't always read the textbook. You might
be having really strong contractions, but they're coming
only every ten minutes. In a case like this, look at the
intensity. If you were to rate your pain, 10 being the
worst pain you can imagine, when you get to a pain scale
of 6, that's a good indicator of real labor. When it's time,
head to the hospital. If you live far away, you may not be
able to labor at home for as long.

WHAT A DOULA CAN DO

A doula can come to your home and help you in early labor. She can offer options for positions and breathing that make a big difference. She can go to the hospital with you and support you through all phases of labor, helping to normalize the situation with her experience, knowledge, and judgment. She can take the pressure off your partner to be good at something he or she has no training in, so your partner can be there for you in the best possible way. She can distract you from pain. She can stay by your side as the nurses care for you. She can be in the delivery room with you and your partner, coaching you all the way through. She can help with nursing as soon as the baby is born. Some doulas also visit you at home to see how you're doing and lend support in the postpartum period. She *can't* check your cervix for dilation (that's part of what the doctors and nurses do). She can't (or shouldn't) be your emissary or advocate in the hospital—that's your partner's role.

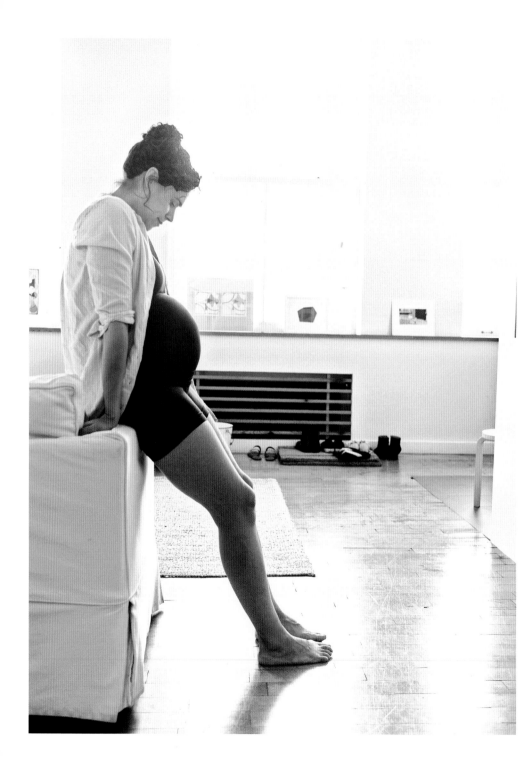

KEEP TWO FEET
ON THE FLOOR

This is our favorite advice for labor. Two *knees* on the floor is fine too. You want to labor vertically for as long as possible, partly to take advantage of gravity. Lying down in labor—which is what our culture does—often doesn't make sense. There are all sorts of upright variations. You can squat with your partner helping to support you. You can put on music and dance between contractions. Once you're at the hospital, you can crank up the bed so you can rest your elbows and head on the mattress while sitting on your birthing ball, or lean on the mattress while standing. When labor becomes really intense, changing positions frequently helps a lot—a doula can be so beneficial here, because she has so many ideas for positions, and so much experience with what works.

IF YOUR DOCTOR WANTS YOU AT THE HOSPITAL EARLY

Your caregiver may want you in the safety of the hospital sooner. If your water has broken, she may want to give you antibiotics. Twenty-five percent of women have Group B strep (detected by vaginal culture at the end of pregnancy). While this doesn't hurt the mother, the baby needs protection. Other reasons a doctor may want someone at the hospital early include bleeding, prior Cesarean birth or other uterine surgery, low amniotic fluid, gestational diabetes, or a sense that the baby is not moving enough. If your doctor wants you at the hospital so she can care for you up close, don't wait. Grab your birthing ball and your support team and go.

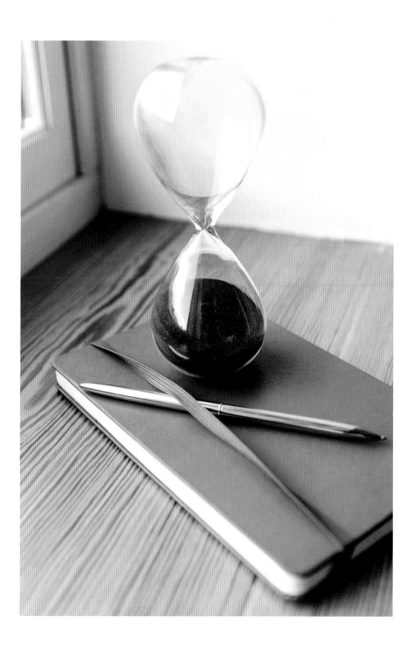

Delivering

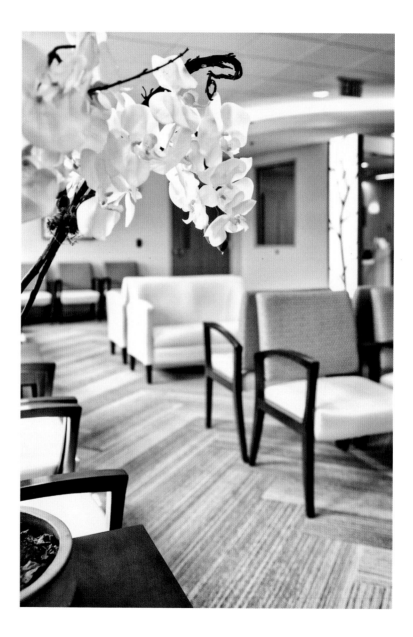

AT THE HOSPITAL

Things are different when you transition into this part of the experience, obviously. Try to keep an open mind and remember that everything that's happening is meant for safety. You'll be put on a fetal monitor and most likely an IV—that's typical. The IV is there in case you should need antibiotics or other meds in labor, and also to keep you hydrated. In your birth plan, you'll ask for a medlock (see the sample birth plan on page 152)—a cap on the IV so you can disconnect from the tubing and stay mobile, with two feet on the floor. It's something the doctor or midwife will need to order when you arrive. If it can't happen for some reason, you can always walk around with the pole (it's on wheels). Keep in mind that the people in and out of your room want good things for you. A spirit of positivity and gratitude will help you relax while those around you do their jobs. You'll have a nice chance to convey this in the tone of your birth plan, and then in small ways (maybe throw some extra snacks in your bag for the nurses). Remember that everyone involved—you, your partner, your doula, the nurses, the doctors, and the rest of the hospital staff—is in this together. Take comfort in the unity of the mission: healthy baby and happy, healthy mom.

EYES ON THE PRIZE

Ultimately, it's the baby who decides how he comes into the world. Even if you have your heart set on an unmedicated birth, there can be many reasons you may need treatment or medications in labor. Sometimes your labor changes in ways we don't expect. Obstetrics is a science but also an in-the-moment art. You're with a practice whose work resonates with you, and the doctor is synthesizing the details of your individual situation as it unfolds. She has her eye on a number of elements and needs to anticipate what might happen next. Her job is to keep you and your baby safe. Trusting her is part of the deal. If you find yourself in the situation of needing an unplanned C-section, don't be upset. Some babies don't tolerate birth well, and sometimes other issues arise during labor that call for surgery. A Cesarean is a solution that brings babies safely into the world. And that's what this is all about.

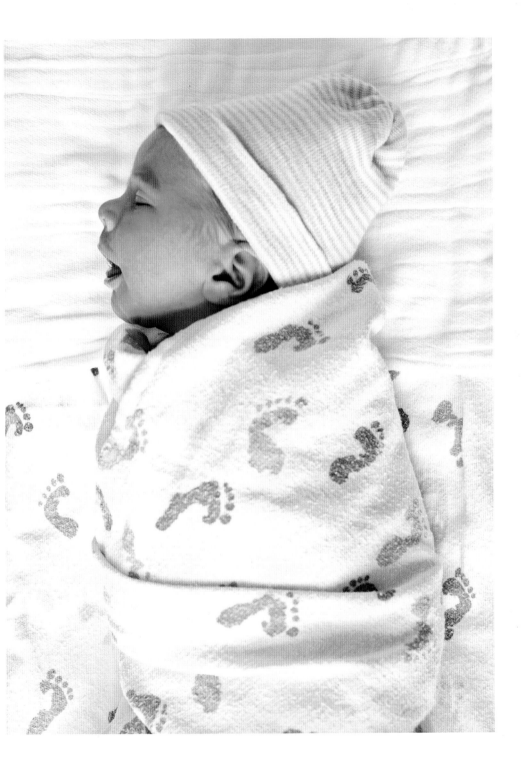

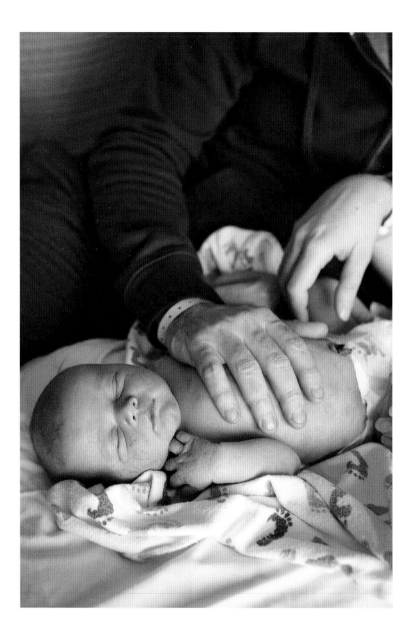

DELAYED CORD CLAMPING

Doctors used to cut and clamp the umbilical cord as soon as the baby was born. Eventually, the medical community came to realize that the blood inside that cord can be valuable: It can increase the baby's blood volume and smooth his cardiopulmonary transition from the womb to the outside world. Now what's recommended is delaying clamping for thirty to sixty seconds and up to five minutes; the doctor watches, then clamps when the cord stops pulsating. This allows the baby to absorb that blood, with all its benefits. We suggest including delayed clamping in your birth plan, but if there's a reason it can't happen, that's fine. As for donating or banking the cord blood for possible future therapeutic use (it contains stem cells)—well, when you delay clamping, much of the blood goes back into the baby, which is great, so there may not be much to give or bank. If you want to read more about this subject, MayoClinic.org has up-to-date information.

SKIN-TO-SKIN CONTACT

The time right after delivery is sometimes referred to as the golden hour. Skin-to-skin contact with your baby during this time is wonderful for bonding, both for the baby and for you. You'll want to have the baby on your body right away, and if you can keep him there for an hour, that's great. Don't be alarmed if you're shaking or shivering right after birth. That's normal. Try to initiate breastfeeding. If you've had a Cesarean birth, this can still be available to you. On page 153 are some simple requests for your birth plan that can make it possible to breastfeed in the operating room soon after a C-section. Some newborn procedures can happen with the baby on you. These include the Apgar, which is an assessment done at minute one and minute five of life, and the baby's vitamin K shot and eye ointment application. Other newborn procedures, like taking the baby's weight and footprints, might be done in the nursery.

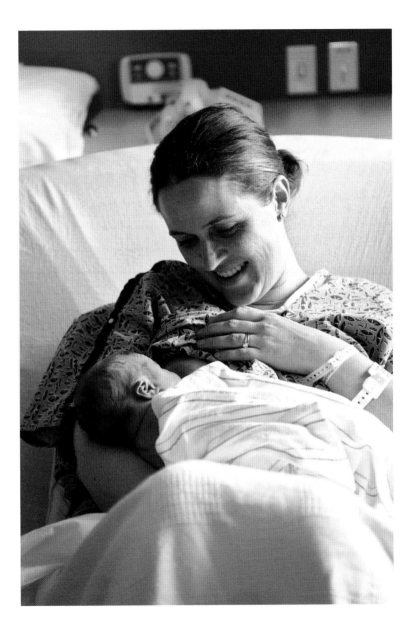

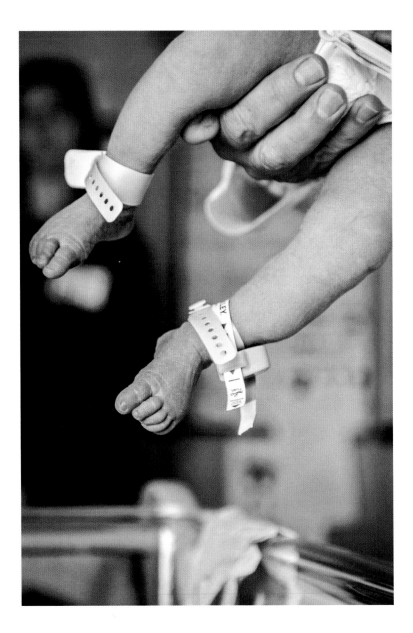

IF THE BABY NEEDS
EXTRA CARE

... that's more important than skin-to-skin contact. The Apgar (see page 192) looks at heart rate, respiratory effort, muscle tone, reflexes, and color of the skin. (It's not physiologically possible for a baby to have a perfect score of ten at birth, so don't worry about the number.) One of the reasons the Apgar is important is that it helps the medical team identify babies who may need additional oxygen or care. If your baby needs help, you want her to get it immediately. Don't feel bad about missing that first hour of skin-to-skin contact. The golden hour is just the beginning of a golden lifetime together. At the soonest moment you're able, put that baby on you. Babies are resilient. Some of the most affectionate and bonded children in our extended families did not have skin-to-skin time during the first hour of life, because they needed medical help. You and your baby will bond no matter when you meet.

PLEASE DON'T EAT
THE PLACENTA

. . . or do something called "vaginal seeding." These practices are something you may be hearing about, but for now, no to both. The placenta is partially a filtration organ, like the liver—a place of waste concentration. There's no evidence that it has any health benefits, and sometimes it can have a high concentration of metals and bacteria. There have been cases of people who've gotten infections from eating the placenta. As for vaginal seeding, well, you may have heard that babies born by Cesarean have a different microbiome than those born vaginally. Passing through the birth canal does expose the baby to good bacteria. But the answer, for now, for babies delivered by Cesarean is not vaginal seeding (the term for swabbing the vagina with a gauze, then wiping down the newborn with said gauze). There are potential pathogens that can be transferred this way. The best way to support the microbiome after a Cesarean birth (and after any birth) is to focus on exclusive breastfeeding. There are ongoing studies being done on vaginal seeding and the microbiome, so stay tuned for updates.

OKAY, LET'S TALK ABOUT HEMORRHOIDS

Hemorrhoids are very common in the third trimester of pregnancy and, not shockingly, also can occur during the pushing stage of labor. Why during pregnancy? Increased progesterone plus extra iron from your prenatal vitamin can cause constipation, which causes straining, which can result in . . . well, you know. And an enlarged uterus pressing on large veins doesn't do you any favors. Hemorrhoids can manifest as something popping out or sometimes just burning and itching. The advice for avoiding them is not revelatory but may be motivating: Eat plenty of fiber to keep your digestive system humming along, drink lots of water, keep moving—don't sit or stand in one position for prolonged periods, make exercise a priority, and don't gain more weight than your caregiver recommends. During labor, well, all preventive bets are off. Treat hemorrhoids postpartum with covered ice packs, witch hazel wipes, soothing baths, Preparation H, and ibuprofen or a local anesthetic spray. Most hemorrhoids will shrink after pregnancy and become a detail you forget in the euphoric recall that gets you pregnant again.

TIPS AFTER A C-SECTION

If you have a Cesarean birth, an elastic support panty will be extremely helpful (look online for the C-Panty by UpSpring). It's just a high-waisted soft, stretchy panty that keeps things from jostling in the area of the incision and also supports your core. Put it on as soon as possible after surgery. If you're scheduled for a Cesarean, pack it in your hospital bag. You'll have an easier time getting up and moving, which you'll be encouraged to do sooner than you might want to, because movement is what helps you heal from surgery. (It decreases the risk of clots and gets your bowels going, which is really important.) If you need some medication to get out of bed and walk, take a small amount; surgery gives you constipation, and so can certain pain meds. Once you're permitted to eat, choose foods that are not likely to give you gas. Continue to wear the support panty for two weeks, then you can switch to a postpartum belly wrap (see BellyBandit.com) for two more weeks. We actually recommend the wrap for everyone, whether you've had a vaginal or C-birth (more about this on page 237). As your incision heals, you may feel a pulling or itching, and the skin around it may be numb. Apply a little Vaseline. It relieves itching, helps the cells migrate and heal, and may reduce scarring.

ARE THEY FISH?

And then land animals? How is it that babies go from living in a sac of water one moment to breathing air the next? This is not a stupid question. The process is another mini-miracle that's part of the grander miracle: When your baby is on the inside, she receives your oxygenated blood through the umbilical cord. Her lungs are not expanded yet—they're not "blown up." The compression as the baby goes through the birth canal squeezes fluid out of the lungs. When the baby is born and we clamp the cord, everything shifts—the baby's pattern of blood flow changes to become like ours. She draws in oxygen—breathing her first breath—then she lets out a cry, and we know it's working.

Nursing

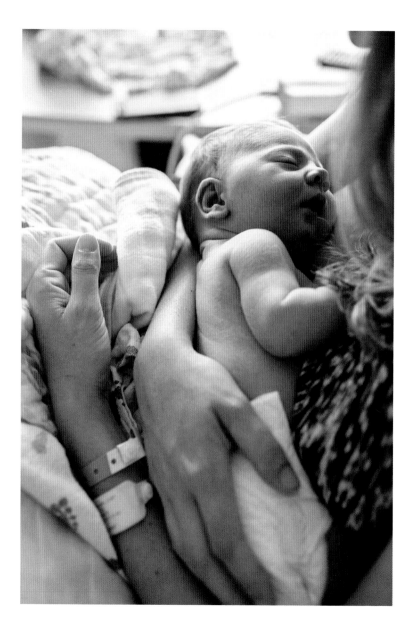

HOW TO NURSE

Your biology is going to help you nurse. Trust your instincts—they're on your side. Here's a quick how-to so you can envision what you'll do: Hold the baby in one arm facing you so her skin is touching yours. Gently brush your nipple along the baby's lower lip—up and down, tickling the lip. This sets off a reflex: The baby will open her mouth into a wide O shape. It may take a minute. Be patient and wait for a big wide mouth—this is the key to a good latch. When you see that big O, place the baby onto the breast with her wide mouth covering the areola—not just the nipple—and the front of her body against yours. You'll feel a latch—a moment of suction—and then she's at it. You want the baby to be facing you, not turning her head to nurse. Once you get it, it's really natural. Support the baby without pressing the back of her head into the breast (babies don't generally respond well to that). If her nostrils are right up against your skin, use one finger to gently depress the breast to create an airway. This whole thing might take ten seconds or a few minutes. When she's done or falls asleep, you can break the suction by putting your pinky either against the breast or in the corner of the baby's mouth.

ASK TO SEE THE LACTATION CONSULTANT

If your hospital has a lactation consultant, request a visit from her after you deliver; she can check the baby's latch and offer some tips. As with doulas, who have been through myriad births, lactation consultants have seen so many babies breastfeed that they know the tricks like no one else—and their wisdom can be invaluable. Have your partner or mom or a friend in the room when the lactation consultant comes—someone who can jot down notes for you and be a second set of ears (you'll be nursing and likely foggy). Even if you have good luck nursing right away, we suggest you use the service if it's available. Some hospitals even offer ongoing breastfeeding support resources after you go home—and some insurance companies cover additional lactation consultant visits; look into it. Sift through the paperwork in your discharge packet (or ask your partner or a friend to) so you're aware what's available. You can also look for a lactation group in your neighborhood. And if you're ever having trouble, you can contact La Leche League International (LLLI.org) or ILCA, the International Lactation Consultant Association (ILCA.org), for assistance and advice.

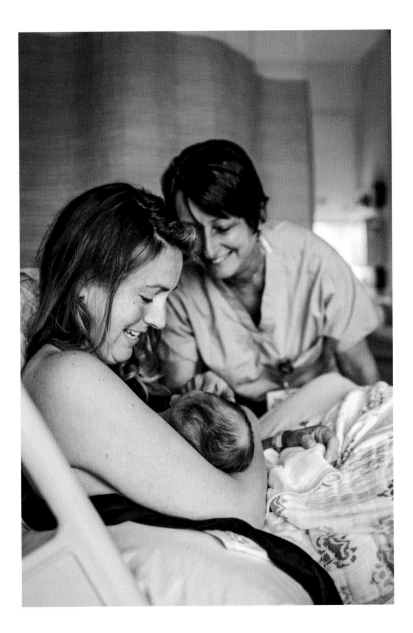

KEEP NOURISHING YOURSELF

Stick with your nutrient-dense pregnancy diet during those first six months postpartum, drink lots of water, and stay on your prenatal vitamin. Your vitamin will help you get enough B$_{12}$, which is important (vegans and vegetarians, we're talking to you), and calcium. Calorie-wise, you'll need 300 to 500 calories more than normal while nursing. If you're exhausted and need a cup of coffee, that's fine (up to two small cups a day). It's trick-ier to pay attention to your own diet while caring for a newborn, but if you don't eat enough, you can start to feel depleted. What you eat changes the smell and the taste of your breast milk, and you may find that your baby reacts to certain foods. If she seems to be having digestion issues, your pediatrician may recommend a tweak—like dropping dairy, avoiding spicy food, or steering away from cruciferous vegetables.

STILL NO WINE

Nursing is an extension of pregnancy—while breastfeeding exclusively those first six months, it's best not to drink. If you're going to have an occasional drink once you've introduced solids (after the baby is six months old), have only one glass at a sitting and no more than two drinks per week. When alcohol is in your system, it's in your breast milk, so nurse your baby before you have a drink, then wait to nurse again—the appropriate amount of time is about the same as when it's safe to drive: two to four hours, depending on what sort of alcohol you've had. (No need to throw away milk—the practice of "pump and dump" is not science-based.) There's also an at-home breast milk litmus test for alcohol you can buy at the drugstore, but you won't need it if you follow the advice here. Keep in mind that alcohol is a depressant, which new moms don't need, and it's caloric without being nourishing.

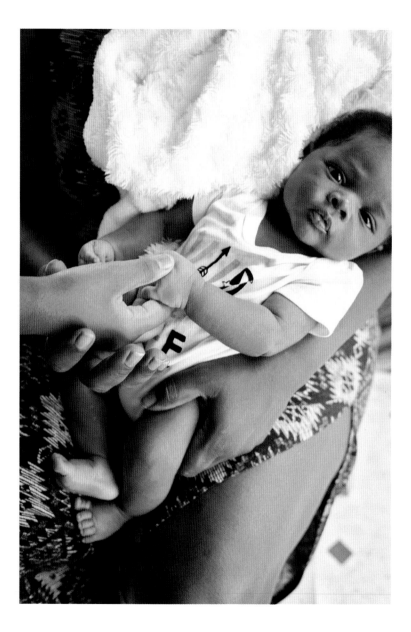

LEAN IN TO NURSING

The first few days of breastfeeding are different from the months that follow. Your milk hasn't come in yet. At this point, when the baby nurses, he's getting small amounts of something called colostrum, a thick early form of milk that's rich in nutrients. There's not a lot of it, but it's all he needs. You might experience some pain on latching in this early stage, not necessarily in the nipple but in the uterus. Latching stimulates the hormone oxytocin, and oxytocin causes contraction of the uterus—it also stimulates milk letdown and facilitates bonding (it's quite a system). So you could get this feeling—like a cramp in the uterus—upon latching. This may go away in a few days or might continue on and off for a few weeks. It's all part of your body's recovery and the efficient circuit that is breastfeeding. It's usually three or four days after you give birth that you notice a change in your breasts; as the hormone prolactin increases in your body, the milk comes in and breasts become firmer, larger, and fuller. This milk is thinner than colostrum (similar to the consistency of skimmed cow's milk), and there's much more of it. Nursing sessions will now be longer. Settle in and enjoy.

FEEDING ON DEMAND

"Demand feeding" just means nursing the baby whenever she wants to nurse (check with your pediatrician). With a newborn, it's the easiest plan. It helps your milk come in at the beginning, then ongoing, it lets your body and the baby's body do what they know how to do. You don't worry about the last time the baby fed and for how long. You don't aim for a schedule. You just give her a breast when she indicates she wants one. Notice signs of hunger and meet her there. You'll be nursing a lot—eight to twelve times a day. But that's what you're supposed to be doing right now. With demand feeding, you don't really need to think. The baby will tell you. In a way, this can be very freeing. At times, it can also be a little crazy-making. There'll be days (and nights) when the baby is at it for hours, sucking and sucking way past the point where she's getting any milk. Those marathon sessions are essentially the baby putting in an order, programming your body to make more milk. Not immediately, but in a day or two. It's a well-designed circuit. If there's a reason at any point that your baby's pediatrician wants her to have some formula, don't worry about being a purist. (You might want to stash a can in the cabinet just in case.)

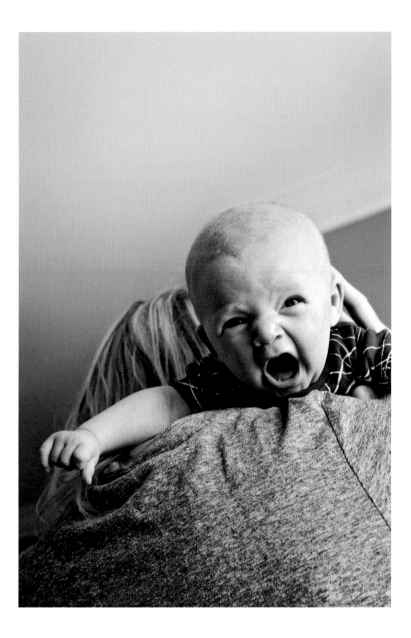

IF YOU HAVE A
CLOGGED DUCT

You'll know a clogged duct because you can actually feel a little hard bump, and it hurts a bit when you touch it. Look online for positions that situate the baby so his chin presses on that clogged spot on the breast as he sucks. This loosens the clog—it's nature's brilliant solution, and is amazingly effective. For relief from the discomfort, get in the shower with a soapy dull comb and comb toward the nipple. Or dangle the breast into a sink of warm water and Epsom salt (rinse off the salt before you nurse again). Then nurse some more. The worst thing you can do for a clogged duct is to stop nursing—because then the breast becomes engorged, and you're at risk for infection. If you have flu-like symptoms, fatigue, or a fever, or if one breast, both breasts, or any part of a breast is achy, tender, red, or hot, call your caregiver. You may need antibiotics for mastitis—an infection that can develop from a clogged duct that's not cleared. Early treatment is very important with mastitis (a delay can land you back in the hospital), so if your doctor wants you on antibiotics, please take them right away. And no matter what—even if you have an infection—keep nursing. It's totally safe for the baby, and it's the best thing for both of you.

WHY DOES NURSING KEEP WEIGHT ON YOU?

Many women hover about 10 pounds above their pre-pregnancy weight till the baby weans. Breastfeeding does burn calories. But the low-estrogen state of breastfeeding combined with a slowed metabolism from the milk-production hormone prolactin may make it harder to lose weight. Take your time and nurse as long as you like, but once the baby starts solids, you can reduce your caloric intake by 300 to 500 calories a day. Once you've stopped breastfeeding and it's time to focus a little more on weight loss, stick with your high-protein, high-fiber diet; it keeps you full and helps stabilize blood sugar, so mood and energy stay even. Plenty of fiber (raw vegetables, beans, fruit, oats) also helps the gut operate more efficiently and keeps you full longer. Always drink a glass of water as a first response to hunger (sometimes the body conflates thirst and hunger). Something to think about if you're planning to have more kids: You'll want to get as close as possible to your ideal body weight before proceeding to another pregnancy. Wherever you are weightwise when you become pregnant again tends to become your body's new set point.

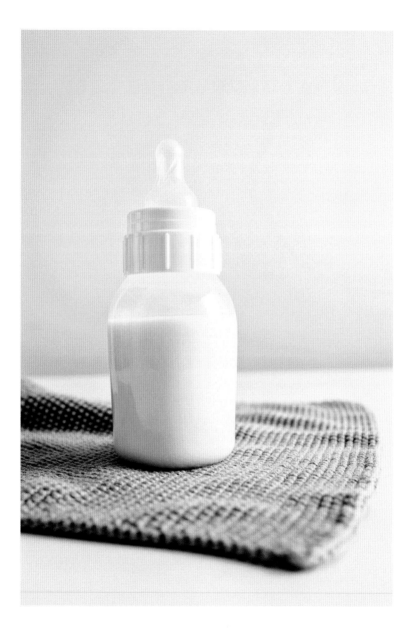

PUMPING: GETTING STARTED

It can be daunting to imagine filling the freezer with milk. Start small. A good way to think of it is to pump a little bit here, a little bit there, so you don't put yourself into over-production. Pump after feeds, not before—there's usually a little surplus. Your breasts tend to produce more milk in the mornings, so for your first few sessions, try right after a morning feed (you can expect 1 to 3 ounces). A double pump cuts pumping time in half, and a pumping bra holds the collection cups in place so your hands are free. Pumping takes a little getting used to, but it shouldn't hurt. If it does, stop and readjust yourself for a better fit. If you know you're going back to work, begin pumping a little bit around week 4. Starting at week 5 or 6, give the baby a bottle of breast milk once or twice a week. Think of this as adding breast-milk-in-a-bottle to his vocabulary. When he recognizes both ways to get his mom's milk, he becomes nimble at going back and forth. These early "surplus" pumping sessions might be ten to thirty minutes; continue a bit after the milk has stopped if you're looking to increase production. Breast milk separates in the fridge (so don't worry—it's not spoiled). For guidelines and advice on pumping, storing, thawing, and using breast milk, go to Medela.com.

EVERY GREAT TIP WE KNOW ABOUT NURSING

- **Take note of early signs of hunger.** Don't wait for hysteria. It's a lot easier to get the baby to latch well when she's not screaming. So when she's fussing and starting to root around for the breast, get in there and see what happens.

- **Let the baby touch your body.** Open up the swaddle, put the baby on you, then put the blanket over the baby, rather than putting the baby over your clothes.

- **Start on one breast for one feeding, the other for the next.** The baby's suck is stronger at the beginning of each feeding; alternating starter sides helps keep things even. There are apps and magnet clips marketed as nursing reminders, but a hair tie moved from wrist to wrist works perfectly well.

- **Don't settle for a shallow latch.** If the baby has a grip only on the nipple and not the areola, it can hurt. Just take her off and try again. And if you see that the baby's lower lip has been sucked in, gently pull it out.

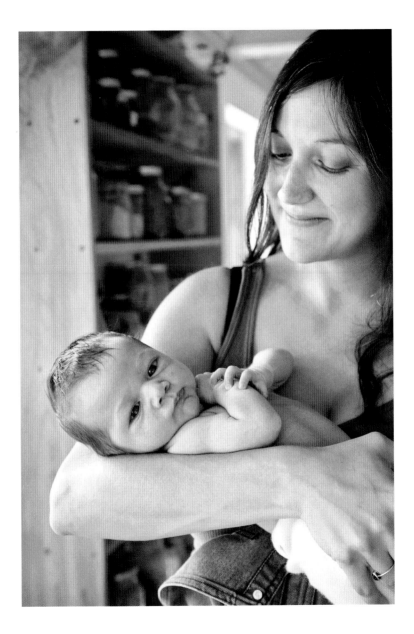

- **Resist the urge to do other things** while you nurse. In the early stages, nursing tends to go more smoothly when you focus on it.

- **Let the baby drain each breast completely.** That's how she gets the high-calorie hind milk (the fattier, more filling part of the milk that tends to stay behind till later in the feeding), which is so important.

- **Alternate cold and warm compresses** if your breasts are overfull. It's tricky for a baby to get a latch if your breasts are engorged (and really uncomfortable for you). You can use compresses or a clean, cold green cabbage leaf pressed against the breast for relief. If you have pain that starts in the nipple and radiates through the breast, use a heating pad; it may be a blood-vessel spasm.

- **Look out for tongue-tie.** If you have nursing trouble, ask the pediatrician to check the baby for tongue-tie, which is common (up to 10 percent of babies have it). It has to do with the piece of skin under the tongue called the frenulum. If the baby's frenulum is on the shorter side, this can impede sucking ability and thus restrict milk flow. This may or may not require fixing but is easily remedied by a pediatric ear, nose, and throat specialist who can use surgical scissors or a laser to divide the membrane.

- **Go scent-free.** Once the baby is born, use unscented products on your body, especially on your breasts; you don't want anything to interfere with your scent. Your baby recognizes your smell, and this plays into bonding and helps with nursing.

- **Wear cotton nursing bras** and cotton tops that can tolerate a lot of washing and offer easy access, either from the top or the bottom. Nursing is so much easier when you dress for it.

- **Wait on the pacifier** until the baby really has the hang of breastfeeding. Ask your pediatrician for guidance before you offer a pacifier at all. (If you do use one, chances are your doctor will want you to get rid of it around six or seven months.)

- **Trust yourself.** Nursing in public can sometimes make you a captive audience for advice from strangers. Most likely, they mean no harm. But don't let them stress you out. What you're doing is right; however you're doing it is fine.

Getting in the Groove

SURRENDER

There's a reason so many cultures have a sacred period of recovery after childbirth—"lying in" or "doing the month" or something else that denotes a stretch of care for the new mother and protection for the newborn. This transition is important, and it's grossly underemphasized in the United States. We're not advocating confinement, but we're giving a nod to the fact that postpartum recovery is essential, and that having a baby does not come with an instantaneous rebound into regular life. Gradually, you emerge from the swirl (maybe this is the word our culture needs for that first month or six weeks—a period when a mom can just nurse and rest). When you're in the swirl, your only job is to foster the growth and nourishment of that new baby (of course, if you have children already, there's more to this, but kids can understand a special finite time and visitors can offer help). Surrender to the swirl, and slowly transition into your new reality. It's a new beginning. Relax—know that you're recovering, and accept that it's going to take some time. Parenthood, if you're new to it, teaches you to be agile—flexible enough to evolve with your kid, and humble enough to know that just when you think you have it all figured out, something changes. It's already changing. Let it.

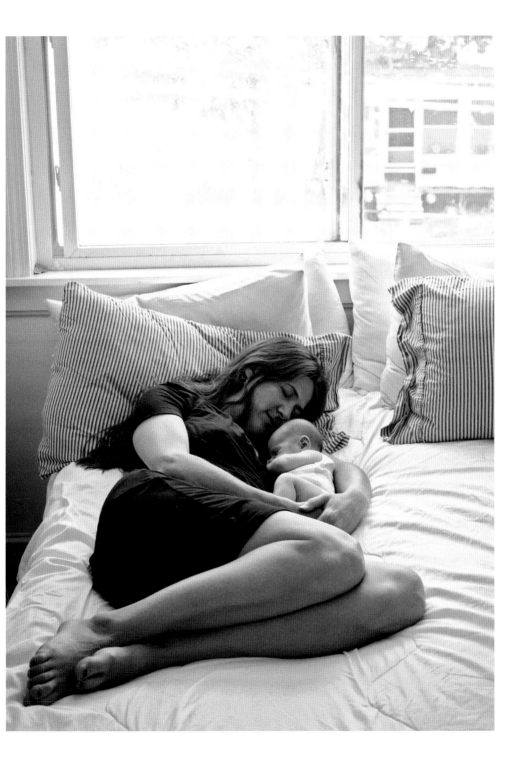

POSTPARTUM CHECKLIST

You'll likely see your doctor when you're two or three weeks postpartum, and then again sometime before the twelve-week mark. You can call or go online to book that first appointment while you're in the hospital. Think of your postpartum checkup as a well visit, a chance to review and reset. Your doctor may give you a pelvic exam and a PAP smear if you're due for one, and will check your weight and blood pressure. She'll see if you're up to date on vaccines. She'll perform follow-up testing related to any pregnancy complications you may have experienced. She'll talk with you about physical recovery (of your abdominal muscles, pelvic muscles, Cesarean incision if applicable, perineum) and emotional well-being. Here are a few things to go over in that visit:

- sleep and fatigue

- pain or discomfort

- sexuality and contraception

- nutrition and exercise

- how nursing is going

- any incontinence issues

- how you're handling all the changes (there's a specific list of questions designed to detect postpartum depression, a PPD scale)
- any pregnancy complications you experienced and how they might inform your self-care going forward

Feel free to bring up anything that's been on your mind (jot it down so you don't forget). Your doctor is there for you after delivery just as she was before.

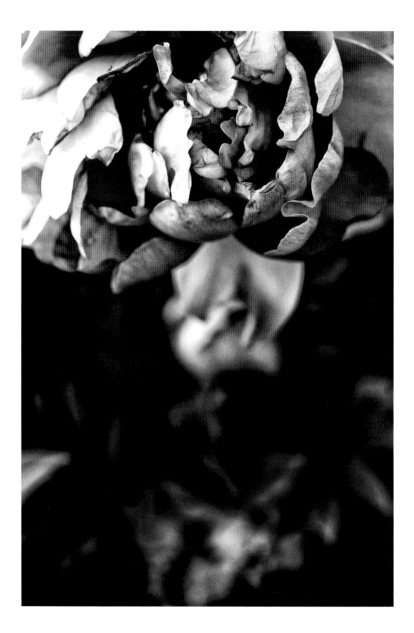

WHY YOU MIGHT FEEL A BIT SAD

Endorphins scale up through pregnancy and are at their highest levels during labor, specifically when you're pushing. They peak to help make labor less painful and enable you to relax. After delivery, hormones and brain chemicals change dramatically. It's biology rearranging your chemistry so you feel protective of the baby and motivated to care for him. But it can also make you feel cranky and tense and weepy. This is perfectly normal. You're worrying for two now. Your brain is fine-tuned to care for this little being—and in fact can become fuzzy on other things (don't be shocked if you find your keys in the fridge). Lack of sleep can make you feel worse, as can perineal or hemorrhoidal pain (use ice packs, ibuprofen, cooling pads or sprays). That's why it's so important to take care of yourself—nap when you can, stay connected, see friends, get outside for short walks—fresh air and natural light can help. Listen to your favorite music. Do anything you know tends to lift your mood. Don't be shy about asking for help. Your partner (or friends or family) may not instinctively know what you need. Speak up to help them help you. Postpartum blues are perfectly normal and usually pass in a week or two.

WHAT MAKES IT
POSTPARTUM DEPRESSION?

If you have a lack of motivation, if you're experiencing apathy and a sense of dread, if you feel despairing and hopeless and these feelings continue past two weeks, if you're struggling with disturbing or scary intrusive thoughts that persist (we're not talking about the occasional flash-fear of something terrible happening), if you're uncharacteristically prone to anger, if you're unable to enjoy life, if you have a lack of interest in your baby—this might be something more serious. Postpartum depression is chemical and treatable. It does not mean you're a bad mom. You need to tell someone how you're feeling: your doctor, your partner, your therapist, or even a friend who can get you to talk to a professional. Don't be alone in this. Your practitioner has tools to evaluate your symptoms, like the MGH Perinatal Depression Scale. Women who are perfectionists or those who had a difficult pregnancy, labor, or delivery may be at higher risk for postpartum anxiety and depression. If you had depression before or during pregnancy, or if there's something stressful going on in other parts of your life, you're also at an increased risk. It's smart to have someone in place—a therapist you're in contact with—whom you can talk to and who'll ask how you're feeling. Don't be ashamed or feel guilty. It might seem like there's nothing anyone can do—that's part of the despair—but doctors, therapists, and medication (there are meds considered safe while nursing, and the field is advancing rapidly) can make an enormous difference—as can exercise and even light therapy. Reach out. As soon as you tell someone, you're on your way to relief.

SLEEP WHEN
THE BABY SLEEPS

This old adage is not necessarily meant literally, but it's a good prompt. Day and night run together when you're nursing a newborn. If you're a first-time mother and can live by your baby's schedule, you'll be more comfortable and rested (the second time around it's a whole different story, of course!). If the baby conks out at noon and three and five and six, take a rest—sleep or lie down or meditate—and don't worry about what the world outside is doing (or wearing). Your own night-time sleep can be bumpy (don't be freaked out by post-partum night sweats; they're just an indication of hor-monal changes). As life begins to normalize, your baby's nap time becomes like gold. Use it to nourish yourself in some way—nap too, eat something, stream a fitness class, read a book, talk on the phone to an adult. One of the interesting adjustments of new parenthood is that you're forced to winnow down—and that gives you a really clear picture of what's worth your time and what's not. When you can, spend precious free time investing in your own well-being.

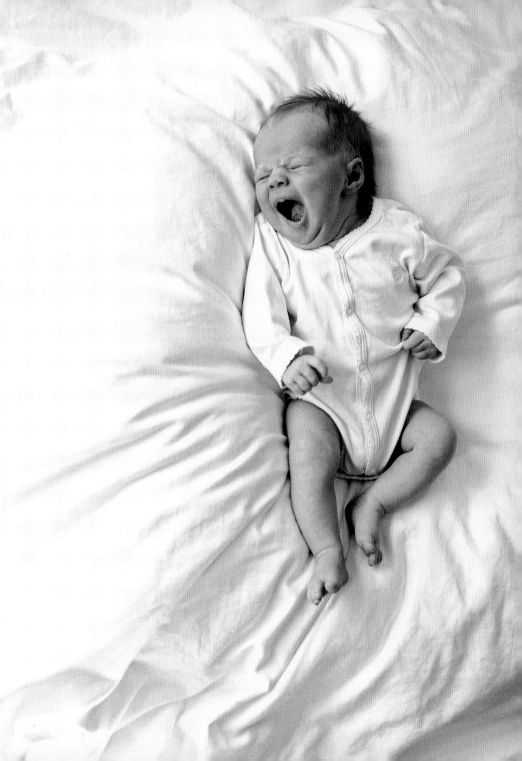

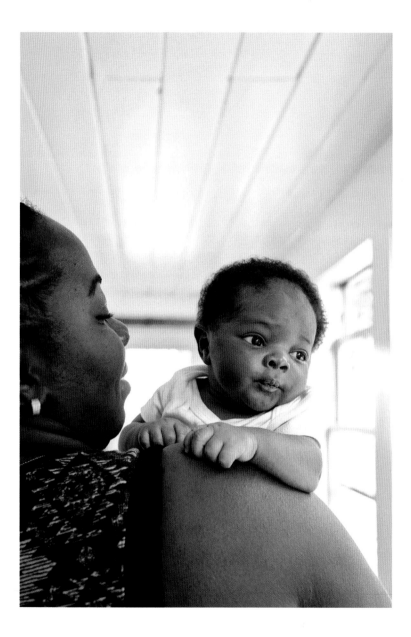

THE FIRST SIX WEEKS

This is a critical time for a newborn—before his first shots, while he's beginning to build up his antibodies—and you and your partner are the protectors. No matter your personality type, you'll need to be a little bit bossy with visitors and pretty tough out on the mean streets. Here are the rules: Nobody touches the baby without thoroughly washing his or her hands. Nobody kisses the baby on the mouth. If someone in the family is sick—even someone close, like a grandma—sorry; see ya in a month when you're healthy. If you have a cold sore, don't kiss the baby. If you have a dog or cat (and we love dogs and cats), it shouldn't be licking the baby's face. When you take the baby out, try to stay in open-air environments. Avoid closed crowded spaces. If you're in a public place, wash your own hands before touching the baby. If there's nowhere to wash, use an alcohol-based hand sanitizer (but remember, simple handwashing is best). When strangers on the street reach out for your newborn's tiny adorable fingers, be a mama bear. You can do this politely. Tell them your baby gets sick easily, so the pediatrician said it's better if people don't touch him. There's really just one rule to follow during this time: Baby comes first.

YOUR PARTNER MIGHT TAKE
A BIT LONGER TO BOND

. . . and that's okay. Partners can feel a little left out in the beginning. They may not quite get it like you do—and they're not supposed to. You are the biological mother, and there's nothing like that. In a way, the partner's role is to protect your bond with the baby. Expecting your partner to bond in five minutes is a little like expecting him or her to know what to do during labor—not necessarily reasonable. Be patient. Dads do experience some hormonal changes, including a decrease in testosterone when the baby is expected—some even experience a type of postpartum depression. And partners can feel a bit neglected, for obvious reasons. Your connection with the baby is very close and intense, and you're nursing all the time. Biology tamps down your sex drive, because nature is supporting nurturing this baby rather than making another. But that doesn't mean you can't be cozy and loving. When trusted visitors come, give them some cuddle time with the baby and take a walk as a couple. Get an ice cream, sit on a bench, hold hands. Talk about something other than the baby. A little refresh can go a long way.

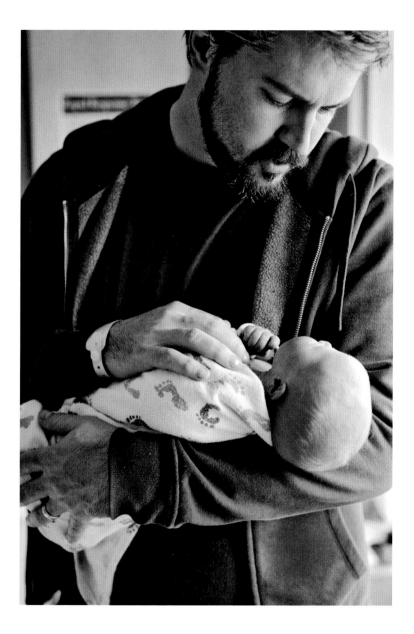

EXTREME KEGELS

Nursing offers plenty of time to sit and do postpartum Kegel exercises; you'll probably feel ready to start by about six weeks. Do as many sets as you like, but at least two sets of ten reps each day. Once you pass twelve weeks, if you want to take this up a notch and your doctor says it's okay, you can add Kegel weights to the equation (search online for a set). They're little slip-in doodads for increasing the strength of the pelvic floor muscles (sets include varying weights). You place one inside, then go about light housework for fifteen minutes or so, and your muscles reflexively pull up, working to hold the weight in place. Once you master the lightest weight, you move up to the next one. It just adds a little challenge and friendly self-competition to the task. Whether you use gadgets or go natural, your postpartum Kegels will hasten recovery, increase blood flow, minimize that pee-when-you-cough problem, and potentially lead to better sex.

POSTPARTUM STRENGTHENING

You can start working on your core again four to six weeks after birth, with gentle Pilates-type exercises like pelvic tilts and planks—no crunches yet. Before that, take care of your body with support garments that keep you comfortable. Even for those who've had a vaginal delivery, a high-waisted elastic support garment like the C-Panty (marketed for post C-section) feels good during the first two weeks postpartum. Then you might want to move on to something more supportive that helps realign muscles while they're healing. We suggest a post-partum belly wrap like the Gabrialla Breathable Abdominal Support Binder (easy to find online). It should feel comfortable and cozy. Try to wear it at least half your waking hours, from weeks 2 to 4 postpartum. A wrap may also help with diastasis recti, that vertical separation of the abdominals that results in a center bulge along the midline—a common side effect of pregnancy (your doctor can ID diastasis recti and offer solutions). For just about everyone, the wrap is a good proactive approach. By week 4 postpartum, unless you're instructed by your doctor or physical therapist to wear the wrap while exercising, you can be done with it. At that point, it's time for your own muscles to take over.

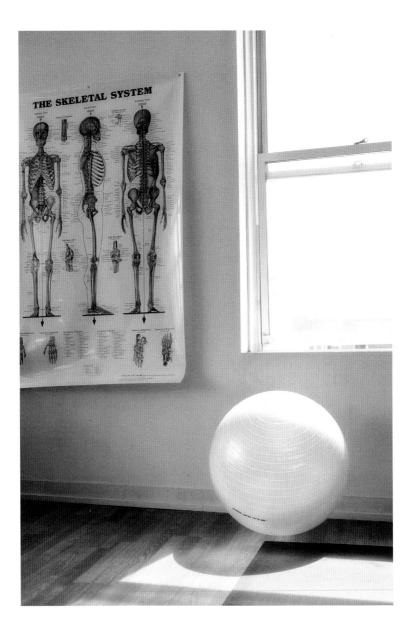

PELVIC-FLOOR PHYSICAL THERAPY IS A THING

. . . and it can make a big difference in recovery. It can involve exercises, trigger-point release, biofeedback, and yes, some internal work. Our patients find it extremely beneficial. Sometimes insurance even covers it. Pelvic-floor PT is effective in treating temporary bladder weakness, which can be a side effect of vaginal delivery, and it also helps with circulation, hemorrhoids, back pain, perineal pain, joint pain, and sexual function. If you had a Cesarean birth, a pelvic PT can also work on softening the scar and helping with abdominal recovery. Tell your doctor you'd like to see a pelvic PT, and she can write you a prescription. We suggest starting about eight weeks postpartum.

SEX AFTERWARD

Your postpartum vagina and perineum are not permanent. The drop in estrogen can decrease blood flow and make your vagina feel dry and fragile, and the perineum may feel numb for a bit. The doctor will likely give you the green light to have sex between two and six weeks after delivery—but obviously, wait till you're ready. Use a water-based lubricant like Sustain or AstroGlide Natural Feel. Take it slow and choose a comfortable position that allows you to control friction (like you on top). Discuss contraceptive options with your doctor at your postpartum visit—IUDs and contraceptive implants are safe and effective, as is the minipill (which doesn't contain estrogen). None of these will affect milk supply. Desire can really wane in the first few months of nursing. Exhaustion doesn't help. You have to be honest about it with your partner. This isn't forever. If you have zero urge, know that there's nothing wrong with you. It's biology. It can be very helpful to talk about this in advance, so nobody's surprised. You'll power through together.

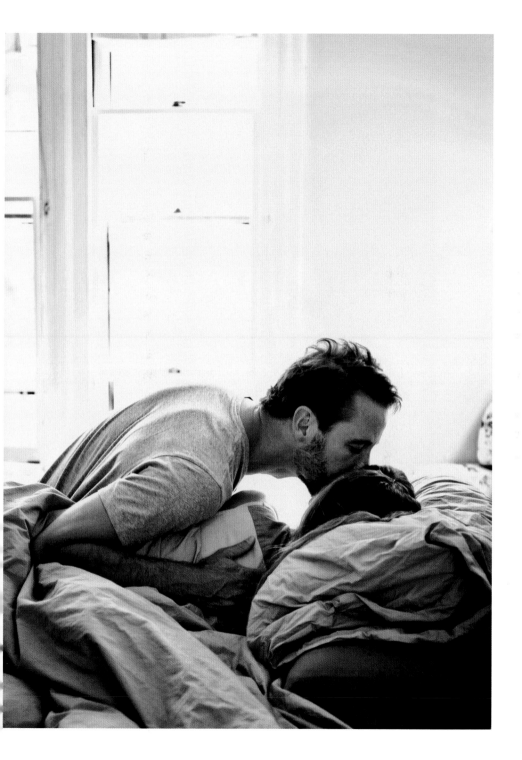

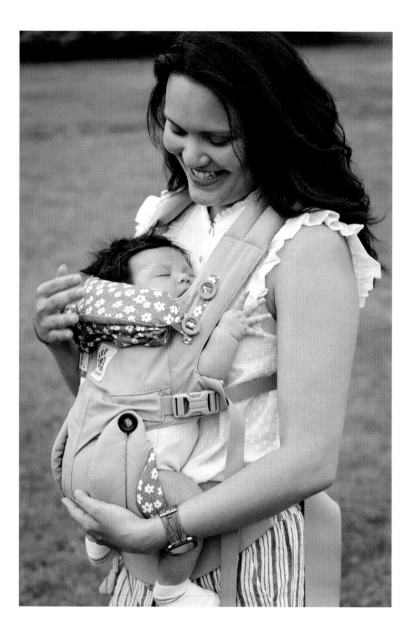

GIVE YOUR BODY TIME

Half the weight of pregnancy is generally gone by six weeks postpartum—this is accounted for by the baby, the amniotic fluid, and your uterus shrinking back to normal size. As for the rest of recovery—the remaining weight, your hormones adjusting, sexual desire returning—there's a sort of natural flow, and you can't rush it. Do your best to take care of yourself during the process, but don't try to speed it up. It's different for everyone. Support each transition at the right time: Start getting back to exercise gently and slowly, soon after delivery. There's a good postpartum fitness program called EMbody (visit Every-Mother.com). Use the abdominal binder a couple of weeks in to bring bones back into alignment and help make lax muscles more comfortable. Do physical therapy or at-home Kegel-weight work when your pelvic floor is ready to recover, a couple of months in. Get the weight off when your body is ready to get it off. It may take about a year, or it may happen more quickly.

LITTLE BY LITTLE

Just as during pregnancy something tends to lift at week 13 or so, recovery comes with watersheds. One of them happens around two weeks postpartum. Whether you're coming back from a Cesarean or a vaginal delivery, around the two-week mark, you may notice you have more energy—and start to feel like your old self again. It's a glimmer of what's to come—a preview of you in your usual strong, capable state with the wonderful new demands and privileges of motherhood. Another marker comes when you get the okay to go back to your regular fitness routine. You remember how strong you are (even if your strength needs building) and what it feels like to be out in the world (even if it's only for a brisk walk). But it's thrilling to reconnect with the you from before, who is now also a mother. Walking down the street with or without your baby, you see the world differently. You look at people passing and think, wow, so many of these folks have experienced what I've just experienced and have a little or big creature at home they would do anything for. It connects you to humanity in this beautiful, corny way. And as life begins to flow more smoothly— and the new you takes root—it's almost hard to believe what occurred over the previous year.

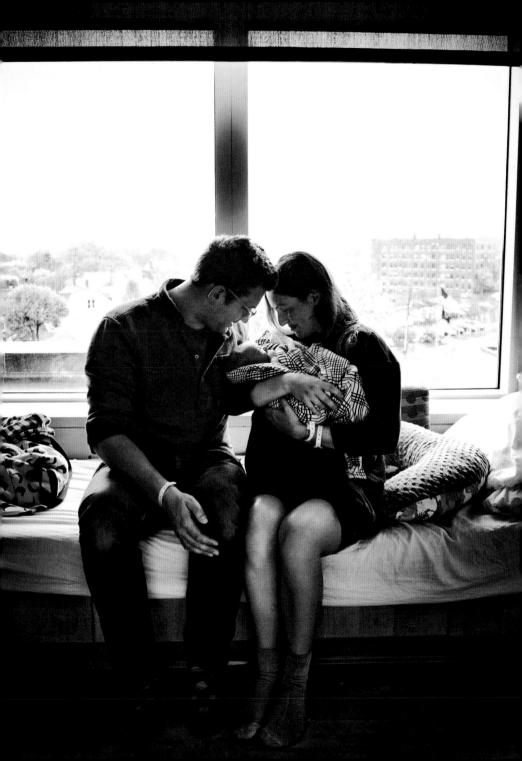

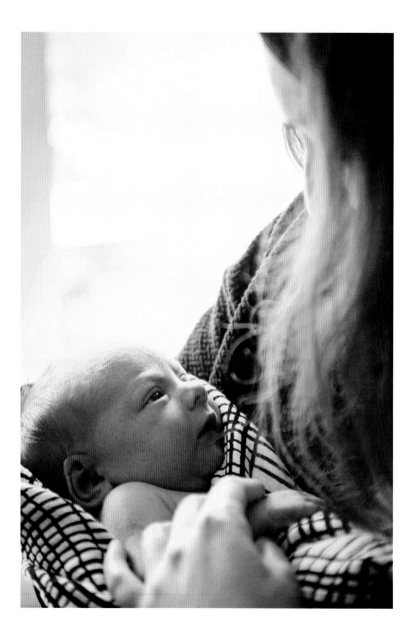

AFTERWORD

When we set out to write this book, our mission was
not only to inform but to bring some of the beauty back
to pregnancy—to remove some clutter and make space
for you to appreciate the profound miracle of it all. We
would like to dedicate this book to all the female physicians who have forged a path through countless obsta-
cles to make a place for us to do what we are so privi-
leged to do today.

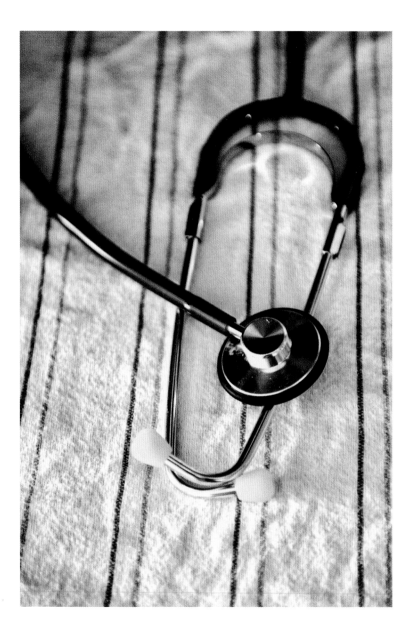

A HELPFUL LIST OF TERMS

Braxton-Hicks contractions: Painless, sporadic contractions in pregnancy.

breech: When the baby is in a position where the feet and buttocks present first.

cerclage: A cervical stitch placed to keep the cervix from opening prematurely.

cervical insufficiency: The inability of the cervix to retain a pregnancy until full term.

chorioamnionitis: An infection and/or inflammation of the fetal amniotic sac, fluid, or placenta.

circumcision: A procedure performed on male infants where the foreskin is removed from the penis.

episiotomy: An incision of the perineum made at the time of birth.

fetal macrosomia: When the baby is larger than average for gestational age.

forceps and vacuum extractor: Instruments used to aid delivery of a baby.

full-term pregnancy: 39 weeks to 40 weeks and 6 days.

gestational diabetes: A temporary condition in which the body processes sugar less efficiently. The risk of developing GD is lower for those who start pregnancy at a healthy weight, gain no more than the recommended amount, and exercise regularly.

Group B strep: A bacteria that colonizes the vagina in 25 percent of women. It requires antibiotic treatment in labor.

IUGR (intrauterine growth restriction): When the baby grows more slowly than expected and is small for gestational age.

jaundice: A yellowing of an infant's skin and eyes twenty-four to forty-eight hours after birth occurring from an excess of bilirubin. It's treated with light therapy.

late-term pregnancy: A pregnancy lasting between 41 weeks and 41 weeks and 6 days.

lochia: The postpartum blood and discharge from the uterus occurring after both vaginal and Cesarean births. It lasts three to six weeks and changes from red to brown to white.

meconium: A baby's first bowel movement, which is often dark green in color and occasionally is passed while baby is still in the uterus.

melasma: Increased skin pigmentation, often on the face, also known by the names chloasma and "the mask of pregnancy." May be found on the areolae and belly (linea nigra).

membrane sweep: A procedure where a practitioner inserts a finger into the cervix to separate the amniotic sac from the cervix. This is a technique commonly used to encourage spontaneous labor.

oligohydramnios: Too little amniotic fluid.

placenta: The organ that brings oxygen and nutrients to the developing fetus and eliminates waste.

placenta accreta: When the placenta and its blood vessels grow too deeply into the uterine wall. This can occur after prior Cesarean or other uterine surgery.

placenta previa: When the placenta is located near or over the cervix instead of at the top of the uterus.

placental abruption: When the placenta partially or totally detaches from the uterine wall prematurely.

polyhydramnios: Too much amniotic fluid.

postpartum hemorrhage: Excessive bleeding after birth.

post-term pregnancy: A pregnancy lasting past 42 weeks.

PPROM (preterm prelabor rupture of membranes): Rupture of the amniotic sac before 37 weeks' gestation and before the onset of contractions.

preeclampsia: High blood pressure in pregnancy associated with other changes in the body, including protein in the urine. Preeclampsia is likely to lead to induction of labor.

preterm labor: Contractions prior to 37 weeks that result in cervical change.

PROM (prelabor rupture of membranes): Rupture of the amniotic sac before the onset of labor after 37 weeks.

Rh negative: A maternal blood type that requires two injections, one at 28 weeks and one postpartum, to prevent production of antibodies that could affect future pregnancies.

SPD (symphysis pubis dysfunction): Pain in the pubic bone and upper thigh worsened by walking or lifting the leg.

umbilical cord blood banking: The collection of stem cells from the umbilical cord after delivery. Stem cells can be used in the field of regenerative medicine.

VBAC (vaginal birth after Cesarean): Labor and delivery in a subsequent pregnancy that results in a successful vaginal delivery after a first delivery via Cesarean.

ACKNOWLEDGMENTS

Thank you to Danielle Claro for conceiving of the idea for this book and for recognizing my vibe from afar and then up close. I am grateful for your grace and femininity, which helped guide us. Thank you to Jaqueline Worth for your expertise and exceptional professionalism as well as your friendship and endless compassion. Thank you to Dr. Mussalli for your expert advice, support, and patience. Thank you to Yajaira, my right hand, for your incredible dedication and compassion, and for helping me help others; your untiring support during this project and over the years has been a blessing. Thanks to my loyal patients for appreciating what I do every day. Finally, to my family and friends: Thank you for loving me just the way I am. —**A. L. S.**

Thanks to our patients—the amazing moms and dads who make this work possible by always asking questions and demanding real answers. Thank you to two women pioneers in birth who inspire me with their enormous insight and determination—physician Virginia Apgar and midwife Ina May Gaskin. Thanks to my three families: my family of origin, Merwin and Toby Worth, who raised six children in a crowded New York City apartment, thus turning me into an obstetrician; my life family, Reed, Emily, and Kate Abelson, who love me; and my work family, Dr. George Mussalli, Leanne Hernandez, Lourdes Alvarez, and Lina Rugova, who keep me laughing. And above all, thank you to the two friends who stood beside me day after day as this book was born: Adrienne Simone, a brilliant physician of extraordinary insight, compassion, and dedication, and Danielle Claro, who infused our words with soul and heart. —**J. W.**

Deep thanks to Winky Lewis for her extraordinary photographs; to our visionary publisher, Lia Ronnen, and our wonderful editor, Shoshana Gutmajer; to all the parents and babies whose images make this book beautiful; to Shira Atkins, Megan Nicolay, and Jordan Elizabeth for modeling; to Jeanne Conlon for loaning us her beautiful home; to the stellar team at Artisan Books, including Michelle Ishay-Cohen, Renata Di Biase, Jane Treuhaft, Elise Ramsbottom, and Sibylle Kazeroid. Thanks to Beth Kobliner, Liz Kiernan, Pascale Le Draoulec, Wendy Odabashian, Gary Belsky, KT Firstenberger, and Alan Stein for their ongoing support. Thanks to my mama, Fran Claro, who did pregnancy so well, and to my father and four siblings and all their little babies (now grown and awesome). Thanks to Muddy Water Café, in Tarrytown, New York, where much of this book was written. So much gratitude to Adrienne Simone and Jaqueline Worth for the honor of this partnership. And most of all, thanks to my kids, Ruby Reilly and Ian Reilly, whose insight, humor, creativity, and high standards inspire me every day. —**D. C.**

Adrienne L. Simone, MD, is a renowned New York City OB-GYN. Her compassionate, holistic approach to women's health care blends traditional Western medicine with current integrative medicine. She graduated with honors from UMDNJ's Robert Wood Johnson Medical School and completed her residency at Lenox Hill Hospital. Dr. Simone has been in private practice in Manhattan for more than twenty years.

Jaqueline Worth, MD, graduated from Bryn Mawr College and Columbia University's College of Physicians and Surgeons. She has been an obstetrician for nearly twenty years and has delivered thousands of babies. Her practice, Village Obstetrics, is dedicated to working with women to achieve a safe birth that meets their individual needs. She lives in New York City with her family but spends most of her time delivering babies at Mount Sinai Hospital.

Danielle Claro is coauthor of *The New Health Rules* (Artisan, 2015), a *New York Times* bestselling wellness book written with Dr. Frank Lipman. She's the former deputy editor of *Real Simple* and was founding editor in chief of *Breathe* magazine. She lives with her family in the Lower Hudson Valley.